SKILLMASTERS

Expert ECG Interpretation

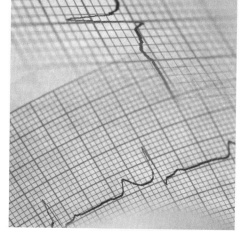

SKILLMASTERS

Expert ECG
Interpretation

LIPPINCOTT WILLIAMS & WILKINS
A **Wolters Kluwer** Company

Philadelphia • Baltimore • New York • London
Buenos Aires • Hong Kong • Sydney • Tokyo

Staff

Publisher
Judith A. Schilling McCann, RN, MSN

Editorial Director
H. Nancy Holmes

Clinical Director
Joan M. Robinson, RN, MSN

Senior Art Director
Arlene Putterman

Clinical Editor
Denise D. Hayes, RN, MSN, CCRN, CRNP

Editors
Jennifer P. Kowalak (senior associate editor); Andrew T. McPhee, RN, BSN

Copy Editors
Kimberly Bilotta, Scotti Cohn, Amy Furman, Dolores Matthews, Marcia Ryan, Dorothy Terry, Peggy Williams

Designers
Mary Ludwicki (art director), BJ Crim (book designer), Lynn Foulk, Donna S. Morris, Kathy Singel

Illustrator
Mary Stangl

Cover Design
Risa Clow, Robert Dieters

Electronic Production Services
Diane Paluba (manager), Joyce Rossi Biletz (senior desktop assistant), Richard Eng

Manufacturing
Patricia K. Dorshaw (senior manager), Beth Janae Orr (book production coordinator)

Editorial Assistants
Danielle J. Barsky, Carol Caputo, Beverly Lane, Linda Ruhf

Librarian
Catherine M. Heslin

Indexer
Karen C. Comerford

SECG– D
04 03   10 9 8 7 6 5 4 3

Library of Congress Cataloging-in-Publication Data

Skillmasters. Expert ECG interpretation.
    p. ; cm.
Includes bibliographical references and index.
1. Electrocardiography—Handbooks, manuals, etc.
2. Nursing—Handbooks, manuals, etc.
[DNLM: 1. Electrocardiography—methods—
Nurses' Instruction. 2. Heart Diseases—
diagnosis—Nurses' Instruction. WG 140 S6275 2002]
I. Title: Expert ECG interpretation.
II. Lippincott Williams & Wilkins.
RC683.5.E5 S496 2002
616.1′207547—dc21
ISBN 1-58255-206-1 (pbk. : alk. paper)   2002005600

Contents

Contributors and consultants

Nancy J. Bekken, RN, MS, CCRN
Staff Educator, Adult Critical Care and
 Medical-Surgical Telemetry
Spectrum Health
Grand Rapids, Mich.

**Christine S. Clayton, RN, MS, CNP,
 CNS**
Nurse Practitioner
Sioux Valley Hospital
Clinical Nurse Specialist
University Medical Center
Sioux Falls, S. Dak.

Julene B. Kruithof, RN, MSN, CCRN
Staff Educator
Spectrum Health
Grand Rapids, Mich.

**Amy M. Obermueller, RN, MSN,
 CCRN**
Assistant Professor
Saint Luke's College
Kansas City, Mo.

Linda Porterfield, RN, PhD
Director of Cardiovascular Research and
 Education
Methodist Hospital
Memphis

**Ruthie Robinson, RN, MSN, CCRN,
 CEN**
Instructor of Nursing
Lamar University
Beaumont, Tex.

**Michelle Robinson-Jackson, MSN,
 CRNP, CS**
Staff Nurse, Intensive Care Unit
Fox Chase Cancer Center
Philadelphia

**Alexander John Siomko, RN,C,
 MSN, CRNP**
Staff Nurse, Telemetry
Methodist Hospital Division, Thomas
 Jefferson University Hospital
Philadelphia

Mary A. Stahl, RN,CS, MSN, CCRN
Clinical Nurse Specialist
Saint Luke's Hospital
Kansas City, Mo.

Barbara A. Todd, MSN, CRNP
Director, Clinical Services Cardiac Surgery
Temple University Hospital
Philadelphia

Foreword

Correct ECG interpretation provides an important challenge to any practitioner. Similar to other clinical skills, practice makes interpretation easier. However, no matter how proficient you are, accurate interpretation can sometimes be difficult. With much information to keep abreast of and limited time to do so, acquiring this crucial skill typically presents quite a challenge.

SkillMasters: Expert ECG Interpretation puts the knowledge you need at your fingertips and helps you meet this critical cardiac challenge. This book is an up-to-date, concise, yet comprehensive reference that serves as an excellent resource for the beginning as well as the advanced practitioner.

This handy manual begins with a review of normal cardiac anatomy and physiology. Next, a chapter on basic electrocardiography gives you key information about the conduction system and its relation to the ECG lead system. An easy step-by-step description walks you through interpretation of an ECG rhythm strip. The clear, concise writing style helps you understand the derivation of the lead system, axis determination, and the effects of various disorders — such as acute myocardial infarction, pericarditis, Prinzmetal's angina, and cardiac hypertrophy — on the ECG.

What follows are chapters covering an extensive array of cardiac abnormalities of rate and rhythm, including sinus node arrhythmias, atrial arrhythmias, junctional arrhythmias, ventricular arrhythmias, and atrioventricular blocks. Each chapter begins with an introduction that describes the class of arrhythmia and its pathophysiology. Then each entry gives important information related to a specific arrhythmia and a quick, error-preventing method to interpret each rhythm strip. For each arrhythmia, you find its causes, clinical significance and appropriate interventions, detailed ECG characteristics, and patient signs and symptoms.

Further chapters provide information on waveform variations associated with electrolyte imbalances, cardiac drugs, pacemaker rhythms, implantable cardioverter defibrillators, and heart transplantation. Included in this comprehensive guide are chapters devoted to 12-lead ECG analysis.

Each chapter in *SkillMasters: Expert ECG Interpretation* gives you access to a vast amount of information, in a cleverly designed format — a format that makes this instructional ECG book unique. Throughout the book are scores of useful illustrations, rhythm strips, and tables.

Special graphic icons draw your attention to important features: *Look-alikes* help distinguish between two rhythms that appear similar and may be easily confused. *Warning* alerts you to identifying lethal arrhythmias. *Troubleshooting* offers tips on solving the most common ECG monitoring problems.

SkillMasters: Expert ECG Interpretation provides a unique way of giving busy practitioners quick access to a wealth of information on reading ECGs. This is an excellent resource for all clinicians who want to verify, update, and expand their knowledge base of electrocardiography.

Kristine A. Scordo, RN, CS, PhD, ACNP
Director
Acute Care Nurse Practitioner Program
Wright State University
Dayton, Ohio

1 Cardiac anatomy and physiology

With a good understanding of electro-cardiograms (ECGs), you'll be better able to provide expert care to your patients. For example, when you're caring for a patient with an arrhythmia or myocardial infarction, an ECG waveform can help you quickly assess his condition and, if necessary, begin lifesaving interventions.

To build ECG skills, begin with the basics covered in this chapter — an overview of the heart's anatomy and physiology.

Cardiac anatomy

The heart is a hollow muscular organ, which works like a mechanical pump. It delivers oxygenated blood to the body through the arteries. When blood returns through the veins, the heart pumps it to the lungs to be reoxygenated.

LOCATION AND STRUCTURE

The heart lies obliquely in the chest, behind the sternum in the mediastinal cavity, or mediastinum. It's located between the lungs and in front of the spine. The top of the heart, called the base, lies just below the second rib. The bottom of the heart, called the apex, tilts forward and down toward the left side of the body and rests on the di-aphragm. (See *Where the heart lies,* page 2.)

The heart varies in size, depending on the person's body size, but is roughly 5″ (12 cm) long and 3½″ (9 cm) wide, or about the size of the person's fist. The heart's weight, typically 9 to 12 oz (255 to 340 g), varies depending on the person's size, age, sex, and athletic conditioning. An athlete's heart usually weighs more than average, and an elderly person's heart weighs less.

HEART WALL

The heart wall, encasing the heart, is made up of three layers: epicardium, myocardium, and endocardium. (See *Layers of the heart wall,* page 3.) The epicardium, the outermost layer, consists of squamous epithelial cells overlying connective tissue. The myocardium, the middle and thickest layer, makes up the largest portion of the heart's wall. This layer of muscle tissue contracts with each heartbeat. The endocardium, the heart wall's innermost layer, consists of a thin layer of endothelial tissue that lines the heart valves and chambers.

The pericardium is a fluid-filled sac that envelops the heart and acts as a tough, protective covering. It consists of the fibrous pericardium and the serous pericardium. The fibrous pericardium is composed of tough, white, fibrous tissue, which fits loosely around

Where the heart lies

The heart lies within the mediastinum, a cavity that contains the tissues and organs separating the two pleural sacs. In most people, two-thirds of the heart extends to the left of the body's midline.

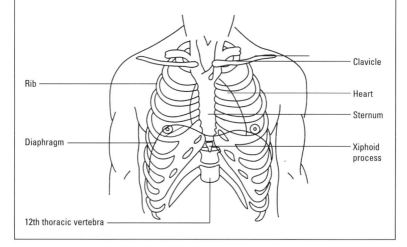

Rib

Diaphragm

12th thoracic vertebra

Clavicle

Heart

Sternum

Xiphoid process

the heart and protects it. The serous pericardium, the thin, smooth, inner portion, has two layers:
■ the parietal layer, which lines the inside of the fibrous pericardium
■ the visceral layer, which adheres to the surface of the heart.

The pericardial space separates the visceral and parietal layers and contains 10 to 20 ml of thin, clear pericardial fluid that lubricates the two surfaces and cushions the heart. Excess pericardial fluid, a condition called pericardial effusion, can compromise the heart's ability to pump blood.

CHAMBERS OF THE HEART

The heart contains four chambers — two atria and two ventricles. (See *Inside a normal heart,* page 4.) The right atrium lies in front of and to the right of the smaller but thicker-walled left atrium. An interatrial septum separates the two chambers and helps them contract. The right and left atria serve as volume reservoirs for blood being sent into the ventricles. The right atrium receives deoxygenated blood returning from the body through the inferior and superior vena cavae and from the heart through the coronary sinus. The left atrium receives oxygenated blood from the lungs through the four pulmonary veins. Contraction of the atria forces blood into the ventricles.

The right and left ventricles serve as the pumping chambers of the heart. The right ventricle lies behind the sternum, and forms the largest part of the heart's sternocostal surface and inferior

Layers of the heart wall

This cross section of the heart wall shows its various layers.

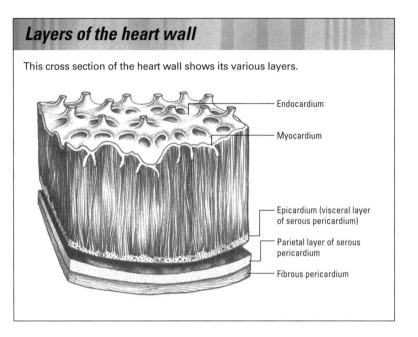

Endocardium

Myocardium

Epicardium (visceral layer of serous pericardium)

Parietal layer of serous pericardium

Fibrous pericardium

border. The right ventricle receives de-oxygenated blood from the right atrium and pumps it through the pulmonary arteries to the lungs, where it's reoxygenated. The left ventricle forms the heart's apex, most of its left border, and most of its posterior and diaphragmatic surfaces. The left ventricle receives oxygenated blood from the left atrium and pumps it through the aorta into the systemic circulation. The interventricular septum separates the ventricles and helps them pump.

The thickness of a chamber's walls is determined by the amount of pressure needed to eject its blood. Because the atria act as reservoirs for the ventricles and pump the blood a shorter distance, their walls are considerably thinner than the walls of the ventricles. Likewise, the left ventricle has a much thicker wall than the right ventricle be-

cause the left ventricle pumps blood against the higher pressures in the aorta. The right ventricle pumps blood against the lower pressures in the pulmonary circulation.

HEART VALVES

The heart contains four valves — two atrioventricular (AV) valves (tricuspid and mitral) and two semilunar valves (aortic and pulmonic). Each valve consists of cusps, or leaflets, that open and close in response to pressure changes within the chambers they connect. The primary function of the valves is to keep blood flowing through the heart in a forward direction. When the valves close, they prevent backflow, or regurgitation, of blood from one chamber to another. Closure of the valves is associated with heart sounds.

Inside a normal heart

This cross section shows the internal structure of a normal heart.

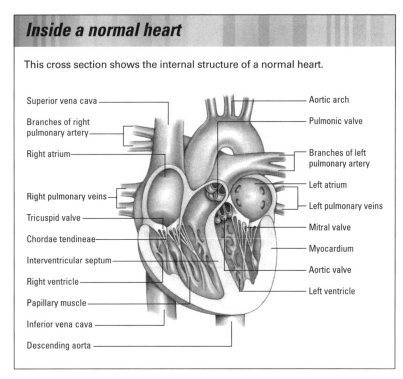

The two AV valves are located between the atria and ventricles. The tricuspid valve, named for its three cusps, separates the right atrium from the right ventricle. The mitral valve, sometimes referred to as the bicuspid valve because of its two cusps, separates the left atrium from the left ventricle. Closure of the AV valves is associated with S_1, or the first heart sound.

The cusps, or leaflets, of these valves are anchored to the papillary muscles of the ventricles by small tendinous cords called chordae tendineae. The papillary muscles and chordae tendineae work together to prevent the cusps from bulging backward into the atria during ventricular contraction. Disruption of either of

these structures may prevent complete valve closure, allowing blood to flow backward into the atria. This backward blood flow may cause a heart murmur.

The semilunar valves are so called because their three cusps resemble half moons. The pulmonic valve, located where the pulmonary artery meets the right ventricle, permits blood to flow from the right ventricle to the pulmonary artery and prevents backflow into the right ventricle. The aortic valve, located where the left ventricle meets the aorta, allows blood to flow from the left ventricle to the aorta and prevents blood backflow into the left ventricle.

Increased pressure within the ventricles during ventricular systole causes the pulmonic and aortic valves to open, allowing ejection of blood into the pulmonary and systemic circulation. Loss of pressure as the ventricular chambers empty causes the valves to close. Closure of the semilunar valves is associated with S_2, or the second heart sound.

BLOOD FLOW THROUGH THE HEART

Understanding the flow of blood through the heart is critical for understanding the overall functions of the heart and how changes in electrical activity affect peripheral blood flow. It's also important to remember that right and left heart events occur simultaneously.

Deoxygenated blood from the body returns to the heart through the inferior vena cava, superior vena cava, and coronary sinus and empties into the right atrium. The increasing volume of blood in the right atrium raises the pressure in that chamber above the pressure in the right ventricle. Then, the tricuspid valve opens, allowing blood to flow into the right ventricle.

The right ventricle pumps blood through the pulmonic valve into the pulmonary arteries and lungs, where oxygen is picked up and excess carbon dioxide is released. From the lungs, the oxygenated blood flows through the pulmonary veins and into the left atrium. This completes a circuit called pulmonary circulation.

As the volume of blood in the left atrium increases, the pressure in the left atrium exceeds the pressure in the left ventricle. The mitral valve opens, allowing blood to flow into the left ventricle. The ventricle contracts and ejects the blood through the aortic valve into the aorta. The blood is distributed throughout the body, releasing oxygen to the cells and picking up carbon dioxide. Blood then returns to the right atrium through the veins, completing a circuit called systemic circulation.

CORONARY BLOOD SUPPLY

Like the brain and all other organs, the heart needs an adequate supply of oxygenated blood to survive. The main coronary arteries lie on the surface of the heart, with smaller arterial branches penetrating the surface into the cardiac muscle mass. The heart receives its blood supply almost entirely through these arteries. In fact, only a very small percentage of the heart's endocardial surface can obtain sufficient amounts of nutrition directly from the blood in the cardiac chambers. (See *Vessels that supply the heart,* page 6.)

Understanding coronary blood flow can help you provide better care for a patient with coronary artery disease because you'll be able to predict which areas of the heart would be affected by a narrowing or occlusion in a particular coronary artery.

Coronary arteries

The left main and right coronary arteries arise from the coronary ostia, small orifices located just above the aortic valve cusps. The right coronary artery fills the groove between the atria and ventricles, giving rise to the acute marginal artery and ending as the posterior descending artery. The right coronary artery supplies blood to the right atrium, the right ventricle, and the inferior wall of the left ventricle. In about 50% of the population, this artery also supplies blood to the sinoatrial (SA) node and the AV node in 90% of the population. The posterior descending artery

Vessels that supply the heart

The coronary circulation involves the arterial system of blood vessels that supply oxygenated blood to the heart and the venous system that removes oxygen-depleted blood from it.

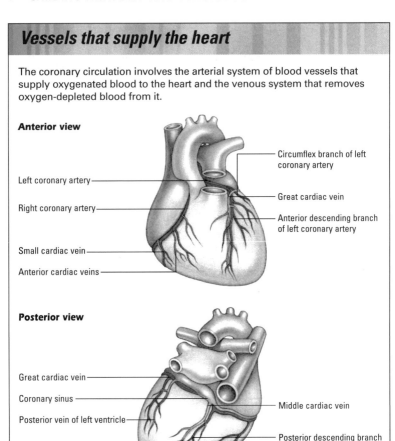

Anterior view

Left coronary artery

Right coronary artery

Small cardiac vein

Anterior cardiac veins

Circumflex branch of left coronary artery

Great cardiac vein

Anterior descending branch of left coronary artery

Posterior view

Great cardiac vein

Coronary sinus

Posterior vein of left ventricle

Middle cardiac vein

Posterior descending branch of right coronary artery

supplies the posterior wall of the left ventricle in 80% to 90% of the population.

The left main coronary artery varies in length from a few millimeters to a few centimeters. It splits into two major branches, the left anterior descending (also known as the interventricular) and the left circumflex arteries. The left anterior descending artery runs down the anterior surface of the heart toward the apex. This artery and its branches — the diagonal arteries and the septal perforators — supply blood to the anterior wall of the left ventricle, the anterior interventricular septum, the Bundle of His, the right bundle branch, and the anterior fasciculus of the left bundle branch.

The circumflex artery circles the left ventricle, ending on its posterior surface. The obtuse marginal artery arises from the circumflex artery. The circumflex artery provides oxygenated blood to the lateral wall of the left ventricle, the left atrium, the posterior wall of the left ventricle in 10% of the population, and the posterior fasciculus of the left bundle branch. In about 50% of the population, it supplies the SA node; in about 10% of the population, the AV node.

In most of the population, the right coronary artery is the dominant vessel, meaning the right coronary artery provides the posterior descending artery. This is described as right coronary dominance or a dominant right coronary artery. Likewise, when the left coronary artery provides the posterior descending artery, the terms left coronary dominance or dominant left coronary artery are used.

When two or more arteries supply the same region, they usually connect through anastomoses, junctions that provide alternative routes of blood flow. This network of smaller arteries, called collateral circulation, provides blood to capillaries that directly feed the heart muscle. Collateral circulation often becomes so strong that even if major coronary arteries become narrowed with plaque, collateral circulation can continue to supply blood to the heart.

Coronary artery blood flow

In contrast to the other vascular beds in the body, the heart receives its blood supply primarily during ventricular relaxation or diastole, when the left ventricle is filling with blood. This is because the coronary ostia lie near the aortic valve and become partially occluded when the aortic valve opens during ventricular contraction or systole. However, when the aortic valve closes, the ostia are unobstructed, allowing blood to fill the coronary arteries. Since diastole is the time when the coronary arteries receive their blood supply, anything that shortens diastole, such as periods of increased heart rate or tachycardia, will also decrease coronary blood flow.

In addition, intramuscular vessels are compressed by the left ventricular muscle during systole. During diastole, the cardiac muscle relaxes, and blood flow through the left ventricular capillaries is no longer obstructed.

Cardiac veins

Just like the other parts of the body, the heart has its own veins, which remove oxygen-depleted blood from the myocardium. Approximately 75% of the total coronary venous blood flow leaves the left ventricle by way of the coronary sinus, an enlarged vessel that returns blood to the right atrium. Most of the venous blood from the right ventricle flows directly into the right atrium through the small anterior cardiac veins, not by way of the coronary sinus. A small amount of coronary blood flows back into the heart through the thebesian veins, minute veins which empty directly into all chambers of the heart.

Cardiac physiology

This section addresses the cardiac cycle, cardiac muscle innervation, depolarization and repolarization, and normal and abnormal impulse conduction.

THE CARDIAC CYCLE

The cardiac cycle includes the cardiac events that occur from the beginning of one heartbeat to the beginning of the next. The cardiac cycle consists of ventricular diastole or relaxation and ventricular systole or contraction. During ventricular diastole, blood flows from the atria through the open tricuspid and mitral valves into the relaxed ventricles. The aortic and pulmonic valves are closed during ventricular diastole. (See *Phases of the cardiac cycle.*)

During diastole, approximately 75% of the blood flows passively from the atria through the open tricuspid and mitral valves and into the ventricles even before the atria contract. Atrial contraction, or atrial kick as it's sometimes called, contributes another 25% to ventricular filling. Loss of effective atrial contraction occurs with some arrhythmias such as atrial fibrillation. This results in a subsequent reduction in cardiac output.

During ventricular systole, the mitral and tricuspid valves are closed as the relaxed atria fill with blood. As ventricular pressure rises, the aortic and pulmonic valves open. The ventricles contract, and blood is ejected into the pulmonic and systemic circulation.

CARDIAC OUTPUT

Cardiac output is the amount of blood the left ventricle pumps into the aorta per minute. Cardiac output is measured by multiplying heart rate times stroke volume. Stroke volume refers to the amount of blood ejected with each ventricular contraction and is usually about 70 ml.

Normal cardiac output is 4 to 8 L per minute, depending on body size. The heart pumps only as much blood as the body requires, based upon metabolic requirements. During exercise, for example, the heart increases cardiac output accordingly.

Three factors determine stroke volume: preload, afterload, and myocardial contractility. (See *Preload and afterload,* page 10.) Preload is the degree of stretch or tension on the muscle fibers when they begin to contract. It's usually considered to be the end-diastolic pressure when the ventricle has become filled.

Afterload is the load or amount of pressure the left ventricle must work against to eject blood during systole and corresponds to the systolic pressure. The greater this resistance, the greater the heart's workload. Afterload is also called the systemic vascular resistance.

Contractility is the ventricle's ability to contract, which is determined by the degree of muscle fiber stretch at the end of diastole. The more the muscle fibers stretch during ventricular filling, up to an optimal length, the more forceful the contraction.

AUTONOMIC INNERVATION OF THE HEART

The two branches of the autonomic nervous system — the sympathetic (or adrenergic) and the parasympathetic (or cholinergic) — abundantly supply the heart. Sympathetic fibers innervate all the areas of the heart, while parasympathetic fibers primarily innervate the SA and AV nodes.

Sympathetic nerve stimulation causes the release of norepinephrine, which increases the heart rate by increasing SA node discharge, accelerates AV node conduction time, and increases

Phases of the cardiac cycle

The cardiac cycle consists of the following phases.

1. Isovolumetric ventricular contraction. In response to ventricular depolarization, tension in the ventricles increases. The rise in pressure within the ventricles leads to closure of the mitral and tricuspid valves. The pulmonic and aortic valves stay closed during the entire phase.

2. Ventricular ejection. When ventricular pressure exceeds aortic and pulmonary arterial pressure, the aortic and pulmonic valves open and the ventricles eject blood.

3. Isovolumetric relaxation. When ventricular pressure falls below pressure in the aorta and pulmonary artery, the aortic and pulmonic valves close. All valves are closed during this phase. Atrial diastole occurs as blood fills the atria.

4. Ventricular filling. Atrial pressure exceeds ventricular pressure, which causes the mitral and tricuspid valves to open. Blood then flows passively into the ventricles. About 70% of ventricular filling takes place during this phase.

5. Atrial systole. Known as the atrial kick, atrial systole (coinciding with late ventricular diastole) supplies the ventricles with the remaining 30% of the blood for each heartbeat.

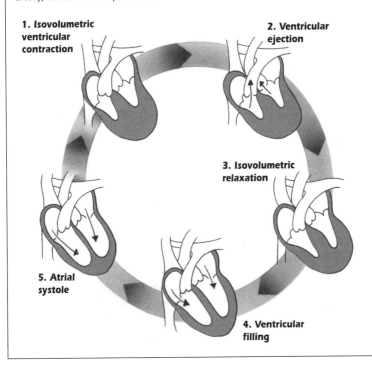

1. Isovolumetric ventricular contraction

2. Ventricular ejection

3. Isovolumetric relaxation

4. Ventricular filling

5. Atrial systole

Preload and afterload

Preload refers to a passive stretching exerted by blood on the ventricular muscle fibers at the end of diastole. According to Starling's law, the more the cardiac muscles are stretched in diastole, the more forcefully they contract in systole, up to a certain point.

Afterload refers to the pressure that the ventricles need to generate to overcome higher pressure in the aorta to eject blood into the systemic circulation. This systemic vascular resistance corresponds to the systemic systolic pressure.

Preload

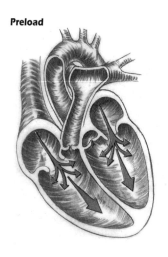

Afterload

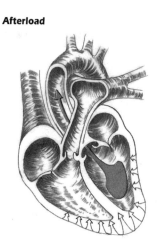

the force of myocardial contraction and cardiac output.

Parasympathetic (vagal) stimulation causes the release of acetylcholine, which produces the opposite effects. The rate of SA node discharge is decreased, thus slowing heart rate and cardiac output, and conduction through the AV node is slowed.

TRANSMISSION OF ELECTRICAL IMPULSES

In order for the heart to contract and pump blood to the rest of the body, an electrical stimulus needs to occur first.

Generation and transmission of electrical impulses depend on the four key characteristics of cardiac cells: automaticity, excitability, conductivity, and contractility.

Automaticity refers to a cell's ability to spontaneously initiate an electrical impulse. Pacemaker cells usually possess this ability. Excitability results from ion shifts across the cell membrane and refers to the cell's ability to respond to an electrical stimulus. Conductivity is the ability of a cell to transmit an electrical impulse from one cell to another. Contractility refers to the

Depolarization-repolarization cycle

The depolarization-repolarization cycle consists of the following phases.

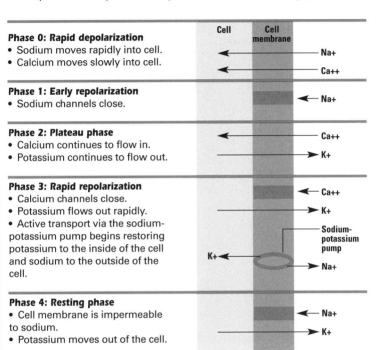

Phase 0: Rapid depolarization
• Sodium moves rapidly into cell.
• Calcium moves slowly into cell.

Na+
Ca++

Phase 1: Early repolarization
• Sodium channels close.

Na+

Phase 2: Plateau phase
• Calcium continues to flow in.
• Potassium continues to flow out.

Ca++
K+

Phase 3: Rapid repolarization
• Calcium channels close.
• Potassium flows out rapidly.
• Active transport via the sodium-potassium pump begins restoring potassium to the inside of the cell and sodium to the outside of the cell.

Ca++
K+
Sodium-potassium pump
K+
Na+

Phase 4: Resting phase
• Cell membrane is impermeable to sodium.
• Potassium moves out of the cell.

Na+
K+

Cell
Cell membrane

cell's ability to contract after receiving a stimulus by shortening and lengthening its muscle fibers.

It's important to remember that the first three characteristics are electrical properties of the cells, while contractility represents a mechanical response to the electrical activity. Of the four characteristics, automaticity has the greatest effect on the genesis of cardiac rhythms.

DEPOLARIZATION AND REPOLARIZATION

As impulses are transmitted, cardiac cells undergo cycles of depolarization and repolarization. (See *Depolarization-repolarization cycle*.) Cardiac cells at rest are considered polarized, meaning that no electrical activity takes place. Cell membranes separate different concentrations of ions, such as sodium and potassium, and create a more negative charge inside the cell. This is called the resting potential. After a stimulus occurs, ions cross the cell

Action potential curves

An action potential curve shows the changes in a cell's electrical charge during the five phases of the depolarization-repolarization cycle. These graphs show electrical changes for pacemaker and nonpacemaker cells.

Action potential curve: Pacemaker cell

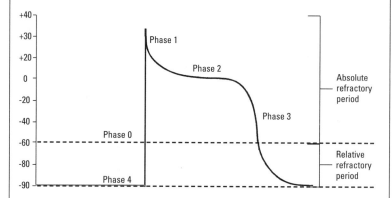

As the graph below shows, the action potential curve for pacemaker cells, such as those in the sinoatrial node, differs from that of other myocardial cells. Pacemaker cells have a resting membrane potential of –60 mV (instead of –90 mV), and they begin to depolarize spontaneously. Called diastolic depolarization, this effect results primarily from calcium and sodium leakage into the cell.

Action potential curve: Nonpacemaker cell

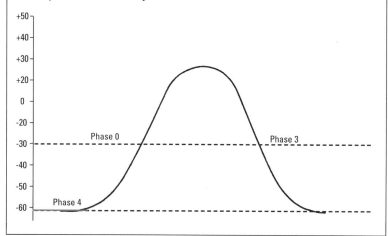

membrane and cause an action potential, or cell depolarization. When a cell is fully depolarized, it attempts to return to its resting state in a process called repolarization. Electrical charges in the cell reverse and return to normal.

A cycle of depolarization-repolarization consists of five phases — 0 through 4. The action potential is represented by a curve that shows voltage changes during the five phases. (See *Action potential curves.*)

During phase 0 (or rapid depolarization), the cell receives a stimulus, usually from a neighboring cell. The cell becomes more permeable to sodium, the inside of the cell becomes less negative, the cell is depolarized, and myocardial contraction occurs. In phase 1 (or early repolarization), sodium stops flowing into the cell, and the transmembrane potential falls slightly. Phase 2 (the plateau phase) is a prolonged period of slow repolarization, when little change occurs in the cell's transmembrane potential.

During phases 1 and 2 and at the beginning of phase 3, the cardiac cell is said to be in its absolute refractory period. During that period, no stimulus, no matter how strong, can excite the cell.

Phase 3 (or rapid repolarization) occurs as the cell returns to its original state. During the last half of this phase, when the cell is in its relative refractory period, a very strong stimulus can depolarize it.

Phase 4 is the resting phase of the action potential. By the end of phase 4, the cell is ready for another stimulus.

The electrical activity of the heart is represented on an ECG. Keep in mind that the ECG represents electrical activity only, not the mechanical activity or actual pumping of the heart.

ELECTRICAL CONDUCTION SYSTEM OF THE HEART

After depolarization and repolarization occur, the resulting electrical impulse travels through the heart along a pathway called the conduction system. (See *Cardiac conduction system,* page 14.)

Impulses travel out from the SA node and through the internodal tracts and Bachmann's bundle to the AV node. From there, impulses travel through the bundle of His, the bundle branches, and finally to the Purkinje fibers.

The SA node, located in the right atrium where the superior vena cava joins the atrial tissue mass, is the heart's main pacemaker. Under resting conditions, the SA node generates impulses 60 to 100 beats/minute. When initiated, the impulses follow a specific path through the heart. Electrical impulses usually don't travel in a backward or retrograde direction because the cells can't respond to a stimulus immediately after depolarization.

From the SA node, the impulse travels through the right and left atria. In the right atrium, the impulse is believed to be transmitted along three internodal tracts, sometimes referred to as the interatrial tracts. These tracts include the anterior, the middle (or Wenckebach's), and the posterior (or Thorel's) internodal tracts. The impulse travels through the left atrium via Bachmann's bundle, tracts of tissue extending from the SA node to the left atrium. Impulse transmission through the right and left atria occurs so rapidly that the atria contract almost simultaneously.

Cardiac conduction system

Specialized fibers propagate electrical impulses throughout the heart's cell, causing the heart to contract. This illustration shows the elements of the cardiac conduction system.

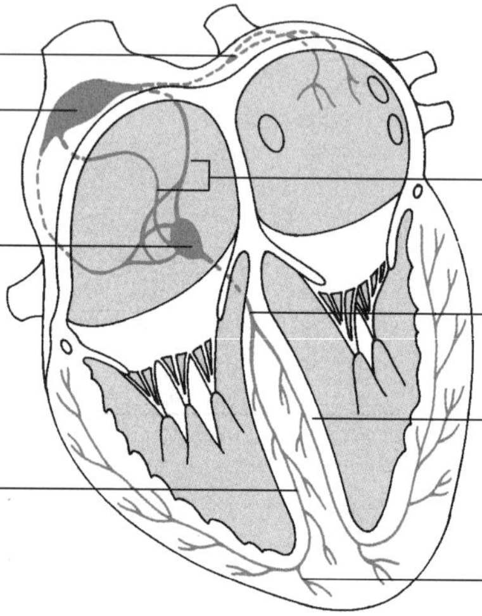

The AV node is located in the inferior right atrium near the ostium of the coronary sinus. Although the AV node doesn't possess pacemaker cells, the tissue surrounding it, referred to as junctional tissue, contains pacemaker cells that can fire at a rate of 40 to 60 beats/minute. As the AV node conducts the atrial impulse to the ventricles, it causes a 0.04-second delay. This delay allows the ventricles to complete their filling phase as the atria contract. It also allows the cardiac muscle to stretch to its fullest for peak cardiac output.

Rapid conduction then resumes through the bundle of His, which divides into the right and left bundle branches and extends down either side of the interventricular septum. The right bundle branch extends down the right side of the interventricular septum and through the right ventricle. The left bundle branch extends down the left side of the interventricular septum and through the left ventricle. As a pacemaker site, the bundle of His has a firing rate between 40 and 60 beats/ minute. The bundle of His usually fires when the SA node fails to generate an impulse at a normal rate or when the impulse fails to reach the AV junction.

The left bundle branch then splits into two branches, or fasciculations. The left anterior fasciculus extends through the anterior portion of the left ventricle. The left posterior fasciculus extends through the lateral and posterior portions of the left ventricle. Impulses travel much faster down the left bundle branch, which feeds the larger, thicker-walled left ventricle, than the right bundle branch, which feeds the smaller, thinner-walled right ventricle. The difference in the conduction speed allows both ventricles to contract simultaneously. The entire network of specialized nervous tissue that extends through the ventricles is known as the His-Purkinje system.

Purkinje fibers comprise a diffuse muscle fiber network beneath the endocardium that transmits impulses quicker than any other part of the conduction system. This pacemaker site usually doesn't fire unless the SA and AV nodes fail to generate an impulse or when the normal impulse is blocked in both bundle branches. The automatic firing rate of the Purkinje fibers ranges from 15 to 40 beats/minute.

ABNORMAL IMPULSE CONDUCTION

Causes of abnormal impulse conduction include altered automaticity, retrograde conduction of impulses, reentry abnormalities, and ectopy.

Automaticity, a special characteristic of pacemaker cells, allows them to generate electrical impulses spontaneously. If a cell's automaticity is increased or decreased, an arrhythmia — or abnormality in the cardiac rhythm — can occur. Tachycardia and premature beats are commonly caused by an increase in the automaticity of pacemaker cells below the SA node. Likewise, a decrease in automaticity of cells in the SA node can cause the development of bradycardia or escape rhythms generated by lower pacemaker sites.

Impulses that begin below the AV node can be transmitted backward toward the atria. This backward, or retrograde, conduction usually takes longer than normal conduction and can cause the atria and ventricles to lose synchrony.

Reentry occurs when cardiac tissue is activated two or more times by the same impulse. This may happen when conduction speed is slowed or when the refractory periods for neighboring cells occur at different times. Impulses are delayed long enough that cells have time to repolarize. In those cases, the active impulse reenters the same area and produces another impulse.

Injured pacemaker (or nonpacemaker) cells may partially depolarize, rather than fully depolarizing. Partial depolarization can lead to spontaneous or secondary depolarization, repetitive ectopic firings called triggered activity.

The resultant depolarization is called afterdepolarization. Early afterdepolarization occurs before the cell is fully repolarized and can be caused by hypokalemia, slow pacing rates, or drug toxicity. If it occurs after the cell has been fully repolarized, it's called delayed afterdepolarization. These problems can be caused by digoxin toxicity, hypercalcemia, or increased catecholamine release. Atrial or ventricular tachycardias may result.

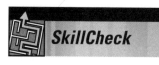
SkillCheck

1. The heart's innermost layer, consisting of a thin layer of endothelial tissue that lines the heart valves and chambers, is the:
  a. endocardium.
  b. epicardium.
  c. myocardium.
  d. pericardium.
Answer: a. The endocardium is the heart's innermost layer consisting of a thin layer of endothelial tissue that lines the heart valves and chambers.

2. Which of the following coronary arteries supplies the posterior wall of the left ventricle in 80% to 90% of the population?
  a. Right coronary
  b. Left anterior descending
  c. Left circumflex
  d. Posterior descending
Answer: d. The posterior descending artery supplies the posterior wall of the left ventricle in 80% to 90% of the population.

3. The load, or amount of pressure, the left ventricle must work against to eject blood during systole is:
  a. preload.
  b. stroke volume.
  c. afterload.
  d. contractility.
Answer: c. Afterload is the load or amount of pressure the left ventricle must work against to eject blood during systole and corresponds to the systolic pressure.

4. Which phase of the depolarization-repolarization cycle is known as the plateau phase?
  a. Phase 0
  b. Phase 1
  c. Phase 2
  d. Phase 3
Answer: c. Phase 2, or the plateau phase, is a prolonged period of slow repolarization when little change occurs in the cell's transmembrane potential.

5. A special characteristic of pacemaker cells that allows them to generate electrical impulses spontaneously is:
  a. reentry.
  b. automaticity.
  c. ectopy.
  d. depolarization.
Answer: b. Automaticity, a special characteristic of pacemaker cells, allows them to generate electrical impulses spontaneously.

Basic electrocardiography

One of the most valuable diagnostic tools available, an electrocardiogram (ECG) records the heart's electrical activity as waveforms. By interpreting these waveforms accurately, you can identify rhythm disturbances, conduction abnormalities, and electrolyte imbalances. An ECG aids in diagnosing and monitoring conditions, such as myocardial infarction (MI) and pericarditis.

To interpret an ECG correctly, you must first recognize its key components. Next, you need to analyze them separately. Then you can put your findings together to reach a conclusion about the heart's electrical activity. This chapter will explain that analytic process, beginning with some fundamental information about electrocardiography.

The heart's electrical activity produces currents that radiate through the surrounding tissue to the skin. When electrodes are attached to the skin, they sense those electrical currents and transmit them to the electrocardiograph. This electrical activity is transformed into waveforms that represent the heart's depolarization-repolarization cycle.

Myocardial depolarization occurs when a wave of stimulation passes through the heart and causes the heart muscle to contract. Repolarization is the relaxation phase. An ECG shows the precise sequence of electrical events occurring in the cardiac cells throughout that process and identifies rhythm disturbances and conduction abnormalities.

Leads and planes

Because the electrical currents from the heart radiate to the skin in many directions, electrodes are placed at different locations to get a total picture of the heart's electrical activity. The ECG can then record information from different perspectives, which are called leads and planes.

LEADS

A lead provides a view of the heart's electrical activity between two points, or poles. Every lead consists of one positive and one negative pole. Between the two poles lies an imaginary line representing the lead's axis, a term that refers to the direction of the current moving through the heart. Because each lead measures the heart's electrical potential from different directions, each generates its own characteristic tracing. (See *Current direction and waveform deflection,* page 18.)

The direction in which the electric current flows determines how the waveforms appear on the ECG tracing.

Current direction and waveform deflection

The illustration shows possible directions of electrical current and the corresponding waveform deflections. The direction of the electrical current determines the upward or downward deflection of an electrocardiogram waveform.

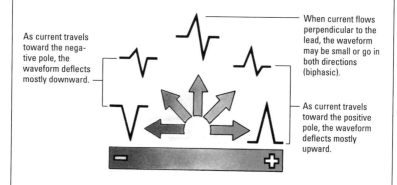

As current travels toward the negative pole, the waveform deflects mostly downward.

When current flows perpendicular to the lead, the waveform may be small or go in both directions (biphasic).

As current travels toward the positive pole, the waveform deflects mostly upward.

When the current flows along the axis toward the positive pole of the electrode, the waveform deflects upward and is called a positive deflection. When the current flows away from the positive pole, the waveform deflects downward, below the baseline, and is called a negative deflection. When the current flows perpendicular to the axis, the wave may go in both directions or be unusually small. When electrical activity is absent or too small to measure, the waveform is a straight line, also called an isoelectric deflection.

PLANES

A plane is a cross section of the heart, which provides a different view of the heart's electrical activity. In the frontal plane — a vertical cut through the middle of the heart from top to bottom — electrical activity is viewed from an anterior to posterior approach. The six limb leads are viewed from the frontal plane.

In the horizontal plane — a transverse cut through the middle of the heart dividing it into upper and lower portions — electrical activity can be viewed from a superior or an inferior approach. The six precordial leads are viewed from the horizontal plane.

Types of ECG recordings

The two main types of ECG recordings are the 12-lead ECG and the single-lead ECG, commonly known as a rhythm strip. Both types give valuable information about the heart's electrical activity.

12-LEAD ECG
A 12-lead ECG records information from 12 different views of the heart and provides a complete picture of electrical activity. These 12 views are obtained by placing electrodes on the patient's limbs and chest. The limb leads and the chest, or precordial, leads reflect information from the different planes of the heart.

Different leads provide different information. The six limb leads — I, II, III, augmented vector right (aV_R), augmented vector left (aV_L), and augmented vector foot (aV_F) — provide information about the heart's frontal plane. Leads I, II, and III require a negative and positive electrode for monitoring, which makes these leads bipolar. The augmented leads are unipolar, meaning they need only a positive electrode.

The six precordial or V leads — V_1, V_2, V_3, V_4, V_5, and V_6 — provide information about the heart's horizontal plane. Like the augmented leads, the precordial leads are unipolar, requiring only a positive electrode. The negative pole of these leads, which is in the center of the heart, is calculated by the ECG.

SINGLE-LEAD ECG
Single-lead monitoring provides continuous information about the heart's electrical activity and is used to monitor cardiac status. Chest electrodes pick up the heart's electrical activity for display on the monitor. The monitor also displays heart rate and other measurements and prints out strips of cardiac rhythms.

Commonly monitored leads include the bipolar leads I, II, and III and two other leads called MCL_1 and MCL_6. The initials MCL stand for modified chest lead. These leads are similar to the unipolar leads V_1 and V_6 of the 12-lead ECG. MCL_1 and MCL_6, however, are bipolar leads.

ECG monitoring systems

The type of ECG monitoring system used — hardwire monitoring or telemetry — depends on the patient's clinical status. With hardwire monitoring, the electrodes are connected directly to the cardiac monitor. Most hardwire monitors are mounted permanently on a shelf or wall near the patient's bed. Some monitors are mounted on an I.V. pole for portability, and some may include a defibrillator.

The monitor provides a continuous cardiac rhythm display and transmits the ECG tracing to a console at the nurses' station. Both the monitor and the console have alarms and can print rhythm strips to show ectopic beats, for instance, or other arrhythmias. Hardwire monitors can also track pulse oximetry, blood pressure, hemodynamic measurements, and other parameters through various attachments to the patient.

Hardwire monitoring is generally used in critical care units and emergency departments because it permits continuous observation of one or more patients from more than one area in the unit. However, this type of monitoring does have disadvantages, including limited mobility because the patient is tethered to a monitor.

With telemetry monitoring, the patient carries a small, battery-powered transmitter that sends electrical signals to another location, where the signals are displayed on a monitor screen. This type of ECG monitoring frees the patient from cumbersome wires and cables and protects him from the electrical leakage and accidental shock occasionally associated with hardwire monitoring.

Telemetry monitoring still requires skin electrodes to be placed on the patient's chest. Each electrode is connected by a thin wire to a small transmitter box carried in a pocket or pouch. Telemetry monitoring is especially useful for detecting arrhythmias that occur at rest or during sleep, exercise, or stressful situations. Most systems, however, can monitor heart rate and rhythm only.

Electrode placement

Electrode placement is different for each lead, and different leads provide different views of the heart. A lead may be chosen to highlight a particular part of the ECG complex or the electrical events of a specific area of the heart.

Although leads II, MCL_1, and MCL_6 are among the most commonly used leads for continuous monitoring, lead placement is varied according to the patient's clinical status. If your monitoring system has the capability, you may also monitor the patient in more than one lead. (See *Dual lead monitoring.*)

STANDARD LIMB LEADS

All standard limb leads or bipolar limb leads have a third electrode, known as the ground, which is placed on the chest to prevent electrical interference from appearing on the ECG recording.

Lead I provides a view of the heart that shows current moving from right to left. Because current flows from negative to positive, the positive electrode for this lead is placed on the left arm or on the left side of the chest; the negative electrode is placed on the right arm. Lead I produces a positive deflection on ECG tracings and is helpful in monitoring atrial rhythms and hemiblocks.

Lead II produces a positive deflection. The positive electrode is placed on the patient's left leg and the negative electrode on the right arm. For continuous monitoring, place the electrodes on the torso for convenience, with the positive electrode at the lowest palpable rib at the left midclavicular line and the negative electrode below the right clavicle. The current travels down and to the left in this lead. Lead II tends to produce a positive, high-voltage deflection, resulting in tall P, R, and T waves. This lead is commonly used for routine monitoring and is useful for detecting sinus node and atrial arrhythmias.

Lead III usually produces a positive deflection. The positive electrode is placed on the left leg and the negative electrode on the left arm. Along with lead II, this lead is useful for detecting changes associated with an inferior wall MI.

The axes of the three bipolar limb leads — I, II, and III — form a triangle around the heart and provide a frontal

Dual lead monitoring

Monitoring in two leads provides a more complete picture than monitoring in one. With simultaneous dual monitoring, you'll generally review the first lead — usually designated as the primary lead — for arrhythmias.

A two-lead view helps detect ectopic beats or aberrant rhythms. Leads II and V_1 are the leads most commonly monitored simultaneously.

Lead II

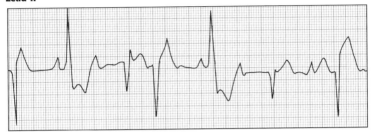

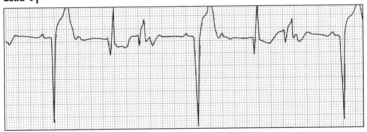

plane view of the heart. (See *Einthoven's triangle,* page 22.)

AUGMENTED UNIPOLAR LEADS

Leads aV_R, aV_L, and aV_F are called augmented leads because the small waveforms that normally would appear from these unipolar leads are enhanced by the ECG.

In lead aV_R, the positive electrode is placed on the right arm and produces a negative deflection because the heart's electrical activity moves away from the lead. In lead aV_L, the positive electrode

is on the left arm and usually produces a positive deflection on the ECG. In lead aV_F, the positive electrode is on the left leg (despite the name aV_F) and produces a positive deflection. These three limb leads also provide a view of the heart's frontal plane.

PRECORDIAL UNIPOLAR LEADS

The six unipolar precordial leads are placed in sequence across the chest and provide a view of the heart's horizontal plane. (See *Precordial views,* page 23.)

Einthoven's triangle

The axes of the three bipolar limb leads (I, II, and III) form a triangle, known as Einthoven's triangle. Because the electrodes for these leads are about equidistant from the heart, the triangle is equilateral.

The axis of lead I extends from shoulder to shoulder, with the right arm lead being the negative electrode and the left arm lead being the positive electrode. The axis of lead II runs from the negative right arm lead electrode to the positive left leg lead electrode. The axis of lead III extends from the negative left arm lead electrode to the positive left leg lead electrode.

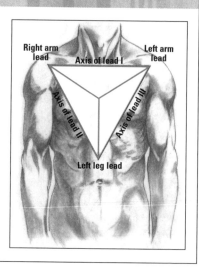

The precordial lead V_1 electrode is placed on the right side of the sternum at the fourth intercostal rib space. This lead corresponds to MCL_1 and shows the P wave, QRS complex, and ST segment particularly well. It helps to distinguish between right and left ventricular ectopic beats that result from myocardial irritation or other cardiac stimulation outside the normal conduction system. Lead V_1 is also useful in monitoring ventricular arrhythmias, ST-segment changes, and bundle-branch blocks.

Lead V_2 is placed to the left of the sternum at the fourth intercostal rib space.

Lead V_3 goes between V_2 and V_4 at the fifth intercostal space. Leads V_1, V_2, and V_3 are biphasic, with positive and negative deflections. Leads V_2 and V_3 can be used to detect ST-segment elevation.

Lead V_4 is placed at the fifth intercostal space at the midclavicular line and produces a biphasic waveform.

Lead V_5 is placed between lead V_4 and V_6 anterior to the axillary line. Lead V_5 produces a positive deflection on the ECG and, along with V_4, can show changes in the ST segment or T wave.

Lead V_6, the last of the precordial leads, is equivalent to MCL_6 and is placed level with lead V_4 at the midaxillary line. Lead V_6 produces a positive deflection on the ECG.

MODIFIED CHEST LEADS

Choose MCL_1 to assess QRS-complex arrhythmias. The equivalent of MCL_1 on the 12-lead ECG is lead V_1, which is created by placing the negative electrode on the left upper chest, the positive electrode on the right side of the

Precordial views

These illustrations show the different views of the heart obtained from each precordial (chest) lead.

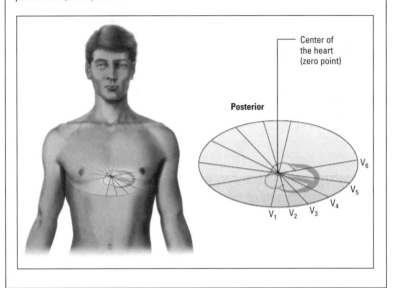

heart, and the ground electrode usually on the right upper chest.

When the positive electrode is on the right side of the heart and the electrical current travels toward the left ventricle, the waveform has a negative deflection. As a result, ectopic or abnormal beats deflect in a positive direction.

You can use this lead to monitor premature ventricular beats and to distinguish different types of tachycardia, such as ventricular and supraventricular tachycardia. MCL_1 can also be used to assess bundle-branch defects and P-wave changes and to confirm pacemaker wire placement.

MCL_6 is an alternative to MCL_1. Like MCL_1, it monitors ventricular

conduction changes. The positive lead in MCL_6 is placed in the same location as its equivalent, lead V_6, for which the positive electrode is placed at the line of the left fifth intercostal space, the negative electrode below the left shoulder, and the ground below the right shoulder.

Leadwire systems

A three-, four-, or five-electrode system may be used for cardiac monitoring. (See *Leadwire systems*, pages 24 and 25.) All three systems use a ground electrode to prevent accidental electrical shock to the patient.

Leadwire systems

This chart shows the correct electrode positions for some of the leads you'll use most often — the five-leadwire, three-leadwire, and telemetry systems. The chart uses the abbreviations RA for the right arm, LA for the left arm, RL for the right leg, LL for the left leg, C for the chest, and G for the ground.

Electrode positions

In the three- and five-leadwire systems, electrode positions for one lead may be identical to those for another lead. When that happens, change the lead selector switch to the setting that corresponds to the lead you want. In some cases, you'll need to reposition the electrodes.

Telemetry

In a telemetry monitoring system, you can create the same leads as the other systems with just two electrodes and a ground wire.

Five-leadwire system	**Three-leadwire system**	**Telemetry system**
Lead I		

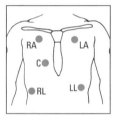 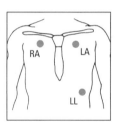 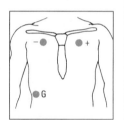

Lead II

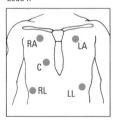 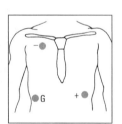

Lead III

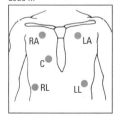 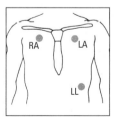 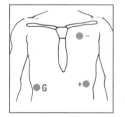

Leadwire systems *(continued)*

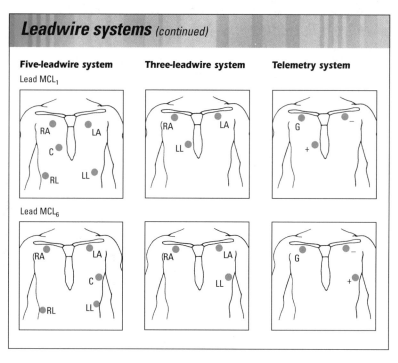

Five-leadwire system
Lead MCL₁

Lead MCL₆

Three-leadwire system

Telemetry system

A three-electrode system has one positive electrode, one negative electrode, and a ground. A four-electrode system has a right leg electrode that becomes a permanent ground for all leads. The popular five-electrode system is an extension of the four-electrode system and uses an additional exploratory chest lead to allow you to monitor any six modified chest leads as well as the standard limb leads. (See *Using a five-leadwire system,* page 26.) This system uses standardized chest placement. Wires that attach to the electrodes are usually color-coded to help you to place them correctly on the patient's chest.

Remember the needs of the patient when applying chest electrodes. For instance, if defibrillation is anticipated, avoid placing the electrodes to the right of the sternum and under the left breast, where the paddles would be placed.

Application of electrodes

Before attaching electrodes to your patient, make sure he knows you're monitoring his heart rate and rhythm, not controlling them. Tell him not to become upset if he hears an alarm during the procedure; it probably just means a leadwire has come loose.

Explain the electrode placement procedure to the patient, provide privacy,

Using a five-leadwire system

This illustration shows the correct placement of the leadwires for a five-leadwire system. The chest electrode shown is located in the lead V₁ position, but you can place it in any of the chest-lead positions. The electrodes are color-coded as follows.

- White — right arm (RA)
- Black — left arm (LA)
- Green — right leg (RL)

- Red — left leg (LL)
- Brown — chest (C)

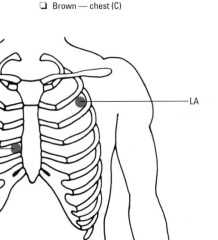

and wash your hands. Expose the patient's chest and select electrode sites for the chosen lead. Choose sites over soft tissues or close to bone, not over bony prominences, thick muscles, or skin folds. Those areas can produce ECG artifacts — waveforms not produced by the heart's electrical activity.

SKIN PREPARATION
Next prepare the patient's skin. Use a special rough patch on the back of the electrode, a dry washcloth, or a gauze pad to briskly rub each site until the skin reddens. Be sure not to damage or break the skin. Brisk scrubbing helps to

remove dead skin cells and improves electrical contact.

Hair may interfere with electrical contact; therefore, it may be necessary to shave or clip closely with scissors areas with dense hair. Dry the areas if you moistened them. If the patient has oily skin, clean each site with an alcohol pad and let it air-dry. This ensures proper adhesion and prevents alcohol from becoming trapped beneath the electrode, which can irritate the skin and cause skin breakdown.

APPLICATION OF ELECTRODE PADS

To apply the electrodes, remove the backing and make sure each pregelled electrode is still moist. If an electrode has become dry, discard it and select another. A dry electrode decreases electrical contact and interferes with waveforms.

Apply one electrode to each prepared site using this method:

■ Press one side of the electrode against the patient's skin, pull gently, and then press the opposite side of the electrode against the skin.

■ Using two fingers, press the adhesive edge around the outside of the electrode to the patient's chest. This fixes the gel and stabilizes the electrode.

■ Repeat this procedure for each electrode.

■ Every 24 hours, remove the electrodes, assess the patient's skin, and replace the old electrodes with new ones.

ATTACHING LEADWIRES

You'll also need to attach leadwires, or cable connections, to the monitor. Then, attach leadwires to the electrodes. Leadwires may clip on or, more commonly, snap on. If you're using the snap-on type, attach the electrode to the leadwire before applying it to the patient's chest. You can even do this ahead of time if you know when the patient will arrive. This will help to prevent patient discomfort and disturbances of the contact between the electrode and the skin. When you use a clip-on leadwire, apply it after the electrode has been secured to the patient's skin. That way, applying the clip won't interfere with the electrode's contact with the skin.

Observing cardiac rhythm

After the electrodes are in proper position, the monitor is on, and the necessary cables are attached, observe the screen. You should see the patient's ECG waveform. Although some monitoring systems allow you to make adjustments by touching the screen, most require you to manipulate knobs and buttons. If the waveform appears too large or too small, change the size by adjusting the gain control. If the waveform appears too high or too low on the screen, adjust the position dial.

Verify that the monitor detects each heartbeat by comparing the patient's apical rate with the rate displayed on the monitor. Set the upper and lower limits of the heart rate according to your facility's policy and the patient's condition. Heart rate alarms are generally set 10 to 20 beats per minute higher or lower than the patient's heart rate.

Monitors with arrhythmia detection generate a rhythm strip automatically whenever the alarm goes off. You can obtain other views of your patient's cardiac rhythm by selecting different leads. You can select leads with the lead selector button or switch.

To get a printout of the patient's cardiac rhythm, press the record control on the monitor. The ECG strip will be printed at the central console. Some systems print the rhythm from a recorder box on the monitor itself.

Most monitors can input the patient's name, room number, date, and time as a permanent record, but if the monitor you're using can't do this, label the rhythm strip with the patient's

ECG grid

This electrocardiogram (ECG) grid shows the horizontal axis and vertical axis and their respective measurement values.

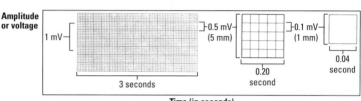

Amplitude or voltage
1 mV
0.5 mV (5 mm)
0.1 mV (1 mm)
0.04 second
0.20 second
3 seconds

Time (in seconds)

name, room number, date, time, and rhythm interpretation. Add appropriate clinical information to the ECG strip, such as any medication administered, presence of chest pain, or patient activity at the time of the recording. Be sure to place the rhythm strip in the appropriate section of the patient's medical record.

Waveforms produced by the heart's electrical current are recorded on graphed ECG paper by a heated stylus. ECG paper consists of horizontal and vertical lines forming a grid. A piece of ECG paper is called an ECG strip or tracing. (See *ECG grid*.)

The horizontal axis of the ECG strip represents time. Each small block equals 0.04 second, and five small blocks form a large block, which equals 0.2 second. This time increment is determined by multiplying 0.04 second (for one small block) by 5, the number of small blocks that compose a large block. Five large blocks equal 1 second (5 x 0.2). When measuring or calculating a patient's heart rate, a 6-second strip consisting of 30 large blocks is usually used.

The ECG strip's vertical axis measures amplitude in millimeters (mm) or electrical voltage in millivolts (mV). Each small block represents 1 mm or 0.1 mV; each large block, 5 mm or 0.5 mV. To determine the amplitude of a wave, segment, or interval, count the number of small blocks from the baseline to the highest or lowest point of the wave, segment, or interval.

Troubleshooting monitor problems

For optimal cardiac monitoring, you need to recognize problems that can interfere with obtaining a reliable ECG recording. (See *The look of monitor problems.*) Causes of interference include artifact from patient movement and poorly placed or poorly functioning equipment.

Artifact, also called waveform interference, may be seen with excessive movement (somatic tremor). The baseline of the ECG appears wavy, bumpy,

The look of monitor problems

The following illustrations present the most commonly encountered monitor problems, including how to identify them, the possible causes, and possible interventions.

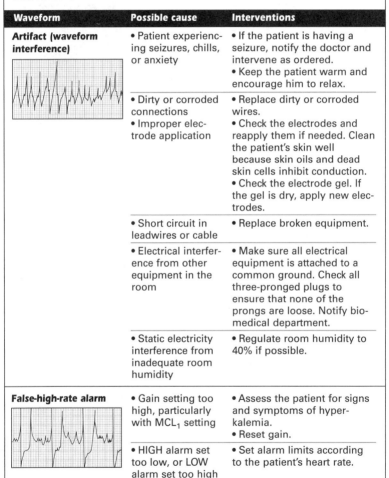

Waveform	Possible cause	Interventions
Artifact (waveform interference)	• Patient experiencing seizures, chills, or anxiety	• If the patient is having a seizure, notify the doctor and intervene as ordered. • Keep the patient warm and encourage him to relax.
	• Dirty or corroded connections • Improper electrode application	• Replace dirty or corroded wires. • Check the electrodes and reapply them if needed. Clean the patient's skin well because skin oils and dead skin cells inhibit conduction. • Check the electrode gel. If the gel is dry, apply new electrodes.
	• Short circuit in leadwires or cable	• Replace broken equipment.
	• Electrical interference from other equipment in the room	• Make sure all electrical equipment is attached to a common ground. Check all three-pronged plugs to ensure that none of the prongs are loose. Notify biomedical department.
	• Static electricity interference from inadequate room humidity	• Regulate room humidity to 40% if possible.
False-high-rate alarm	• Gain setting too high, particularly with MCL$_1$ setting	• Assess the patient for signs and symptoms of hyperkalemia. • Reset gain.
	• HIGH alarm set too low, or LOW alarm set too high	• Set alarm limits according to the patient's heart rate.

(continued)

The look of monitor problems (continued)

Waveform	Possible cause	Interventions
Weak signals	• Improper electrode application	• Reapply the electrodes.
	• QRS complex too small to register	• Reset gain so that the height of the complex is greater than 1 mV. • Try monitoring the patient on another lead.
	• Wire or cable failure	• Replace any faulty wires or cables.
Wandering baseline	• Patient restless	• Encourage the patient to relax.
	• Chest wall movement during respiration	• Make sure that tension on the cable isn't pulling the electrode away from the patient's body.
	• Improper electrode application; electrode positioned over bone	• Reposition improperly placed electrodes.
Fuzzy baseline (electrical interference)	• Electrical interference from other equipment in the room	• Ensure that all electrical equipment is attached to a common ground. • Check all three-pronged plugs to make sure none of the prongs are loose.
	• Improper grounding of the patient's bed	• Ensure that the bed ground is attached to the room's common ground.
	• Electrode malfunction	• Replace the electrodes.
Baseline (no waveform)	• Improper electrode placement (perpendicular to axis of heart)	• Reposition improperly placed electrodes.
	• Electrode disconnected	• Check if electrodes are disconnected.
	• Dry electrode gel	• Check electrode gel. If the gel is dry, apply new electrodes.
	• Wire or cable failure	• Replace any faulty wires or cables.

or tremulous. Dry electrodes may also cause this problem due to poor contact.

Electrical interference or AC interference, also called 60-cycle interference, is caused by electrical power leakage. It may also occur due to interference from other room equipment or improperly grounded equipment. As a result, the lost current pulses at a rate of 60 cycles per second. This interference appears on the ECG as a baseline that is thick and unreadable.

A wandering baseline undulates, meaning that all waveforms are present but the baseline isn't stationary. Movement of the chest wall during respiration, poor electrode placement, or poor electrode contact usually causes this problem.

Faulty equipment, such as broken leadwires and cables, also can cause monitoring problems. Excessively worn equipment can cause improper grounding, putting the patient at risk for accidental shock.

Be aware that some types of artifact resemble arrhythmias and the monitor will interpret them as such. For instance, the monitor may sense a small movement, such as the patient brushing his teeth, as a potentially lethal ventricular tachycardia. So remember to treat the patient, not the monitor. The more familiar you become with your unit's monitoring system — and with your patient — the more quickly you can recognize and interpret problems and act appropriately.

Analyzing a rhythm strip

An ECG complex represents the electrical events occurring in one cardiac cycle. A complex consists of five waveforms labeled with the letters P, Q, R, S, and T. The middle three letters — Q, R, and S — are referred to as a unit, the QRS complex. ECG tracings represent the conduction of electrical impulses from the atria to the ventricles. (See *ECG waveform components,* page 32.)

P WAVE

The P wave is the first component of a normal ECG waveform. It represents atrial depolarization or conduction of an electrical impulse through the atria. When evaluating a P wave, look closely at its characteristics, especially its location, configuration, and deflection. A normal P wave has the following characteristics:

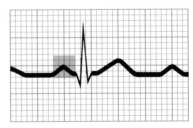

- *location:* precedes the QRS complex
- *amplitude:* 2 to 3 mm high
- *duration:* 0.06 to 0.12 second
- *configuration:* usually rounded and upright
- *deflection:* positive or upright in leads I, II, aV_F, and V_2 to V_6; usually positive but may vary in leads III and aV_L; negative or inverted in lead aV_R; biphasic or variable in lead V_1.

ECG waveform components

This illustration shows the components of a normal ECG waveform.

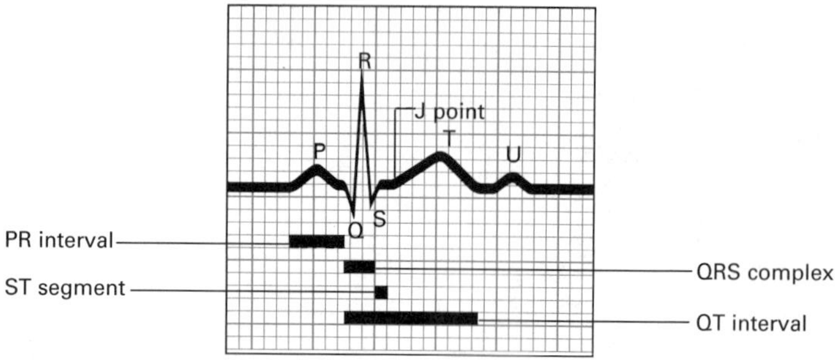

If the deflection and configuration of a P wave are normal — for example, if the P wave is upright in lead II and is rounded and smooth — and if the P wave precedes each QRS complex, you can assume that this electrical impulse originated in the sinoatrial (SA) node. The atria start to contract partway through the P wave, but you won't see this on the ECG. Remember, the ECG records electrical activity only, not mechanical activity or contraction.

Peaked, notched, or enlarged P waves may represent atrial hypertrophy or enlargement associated with chronic obstructive pulmonary disease, pulmonary emboli, valvular disease, or heart failure. Inverted P waves may signify retrograde or reverse conduction from the atrioventricular (AV) junction toward the atria. Whenever an upright sinus P wave becomes inverted, consider retrograde or reverse conduction as possible conditions.

Varying P waves indicate that the impulse may be coming from different sites, as with a wandering pacemaker rhythm, irritable atrial tissue, or damage near the SA node. Absent P waves may signify conduction by a route other than the SA node, as with a junctional or atrial fibrillation rhythm. When a P wave doesn't precede the QRS complex, complete heart block may be present.

PR INTERVAL

The PR interval tracks the atrial impulse from the atria through the AV node, bundle of His, and right and left bundle branches. When evaluating a PR interval, look especially at its duration. Changes in the PR interval indicate an altered impulse formation or a conduction delay, as seen in AV block. A normal PR interval has the following characteristics (amplitude, configuration, and deflection aren't measured):

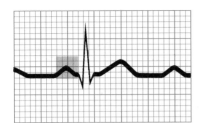

- *location:* from the beginning of the P wave to the beginning of the QRS complex
- *duration:* 0.12 to 0.20 second.

Short PR intervals (less than 0.12 second) indicate that the impulse originated somewhere other than the SA node. This variation is associated with junctional arrhythmias and preexcitation syndromes. Prolonged PR intervals (greater than 0.20 second) may represent a conduction delay through the atria or AV junction due to digoxin toxicity or heart block — slowing related to ischemia or conduction tissue disease.

QRS COMPLEX

The QRS complex follows the P wave and represents depolarization of the ventricles, or impulse conduction. Immediately after the ventricles depolarize, as represented by the QRS complex, they contract. That contraction ejects blood from the ventricles and pumps it through the arteries, creating a pulse.

Whenever you're monitoring cardiac rhythm, remember that the waveform you see represents the heart's electrical activity only. It doesn't guarantee a mechanical contraction of the heart and a subsequent pulse. The contraction could be weak, as happens with premature ventricular contractions, or absent, as happens with pulseless electrical ac-

tivity. So before you treat the strip, check the patient.

Pay special attention to the duration and configuration when evaluating a QRS complex. A normal complex has the following characteristics:

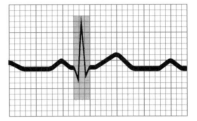

- *location:* follows the PR interval
- *amplitude:* 5 to 30 mm high, but differs for each lead used
- *duration:* 0.06 to 0.10 second, or half of the PR interval. Duration is measured from the beginning of the Q wave to the end of the S wave or from the beginning of the R wave if the Q wave is absent.
- *configuration:* consists of the Q wave (the first negative deflection, or deflection below the baseline, after the P wave), the R wave (the first positive deflection after the Q wave), and the S wave (the first negative deflection after the R wave). You may not always see all three waves. The ventricles depolarize quickly, minimizing contact time between the stylus and the ECG paper, so the QRS complex typically appears thinner than other ECG components. It may also look different in each lead. (See *QRS waveform variety,* page 34.)
- *deflection:* positive (with most of the complex above the baseline) in leads I, II, III, aV_L, aV_F, and V_4 to V_6 and negative in leads aV_R and V_1 to V_3.

Remember that the QRS complex represents intraventricular conduction time. That's why identifying and cor-

QRS waveform variety

The illustrations below show the various configurations of QRS complexes. When documenting the QRS complex, use uppercase letters to indicate a wave with a normal or high amplitude (greater than 5 mm) and lowercase letters to indicate one with a low amplitude (less than 5 mm).

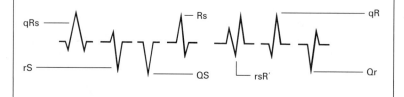

rectly interpreting it is so crucial. If no P wave appears with the QRS complex, then the impulse may have originated in the ventricles, indicating a ventricular arrhythmia.

Deep, wide Q waves may represent MI. In this case, the Q wave amplitude (depth) is greater than or equal to 25% of the height of the succeeding R-wave, or the duration of the Q wave is 0.04 second or more. A notched R wave may signify a bundle-branch block. A widened QRS complex (greater than 0.12 second) may signify a ventricular conduction delay. A missing QRS complex may indicate AV block or ventricular standstill.

ST SEGMENT

The ST segment represents the end of ventricular conduction or depolarization and the beginning of ventricular recovery or repolarization. The point that marks the end of the QRS complex and the beginning of the ST segment is known as the J point.

Pay special attention to the deflection of an ST segment. A normal ST segment has the following characteristics (amplitude, duration, and configuration aren't observed):

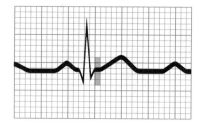

- *location:* extends from the S wave to the beginning of the T wave
- *deflection:* usually isoelectric (neither positive nor negative); may vary from –0.5 to +1 mm in some precordial leads.

A change in the ST segment may indicate myocardial injury or ischemia. An ST segment may become either elevated or depressed. (See *Changes in the ST segment.*)

T WAVE

The peak of the T wave represents the relative refractory period of repolarization or ventricular recovery. When evaluating a T wave, look at the amplitude, configuration, and deflection.

Changes in the ST segment

Closely monitoring the ST segment on a patient's electrocardiogram can help you detect ischemia or injury before infarction develops.

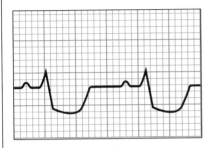

ST-segment depression
An ST segment is considered depressed when it is 0.5 mm or more below the baseline. A depressed ST segment may indicate myocardial ischemia or digoxin toxicity.

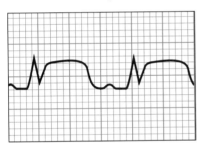

ST-segment elevation
An ST segment is considered elevated when it is 1 mm or more above the baseline. An elevated ST segment may indicate myocardial injury.

Normal T waves have the following characteristics (duration isn't measured):

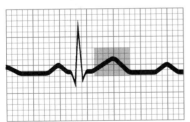

■ *location:* follows the S wave
■ *amplitude:* 0.5 mm in leads I, II, and III and up to 10 mm in the precordial leads
■ *configuration:* typically rounded and smooth

■ *deflection:* usually positive or upright in leads I, II, and V_3 to V_6; inverted in lead aV_R; variable in all other leads.

The T wave's peak represents the relative refractory period of ventricular repolarization, a period during which cells are especially vulnerable to extra stimuli. Bumps in a T wave may indicate that a P wave is hidden in it. If a P wave is hidden, atrial depolarization has occurred, the impulse having originated at a site above the ventricles.

Tall, peaked, or "tented" T waves may indicate myocardial injury or electrolyte imbalances such as hyperkalemia. Inverted T waves in leads I, II, or V_3 through V_6 may represent myocardial ischemia. Heavily notched or pointed T waves in an adult may mean pericarditis in adults.

QT INTERVAL

The QT interval measures the time needed for ventricular depolarization and repolarization. The length of the QT interval varies according to heart rate. The faster the heart rate, the shorter the QT interval. When checking the QT interval, look closely at the duration.

A normal QT interval has the following characteristics (amplitude, configuration, and deflection aren't observed):

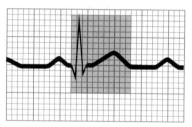

- *location:* extends from the beginning of the QRS complex to the end of the T wave
- *duration:* varies according to age, sex, and heart rate; usually lasts from 0.36 to 0.44 second; shouldn't be greater than half the distance between the two consecutive R waves (called the R-R interval) when the rhythm is regular.

The QT interval measures the time needed for ventricular depolarization and repolarization. Prolonged QT intervals indicate that ventricular repolarization time is slowed, meaning that the relative refractory or vulnerable period of the cardiac cycle is longer.

This variation is also associated with certain medications such as Class I an-

tiarrhythmics. Prolonged QT syndrome is a congenital conduction-system defect present in certain families. Short QT intervals may result from digoxin toxicity or electrolyte imbalances such as hypercalcemia.

U WAVE

The U wave represents repolarization of the His-Purkinje system or ventricular conduction fibers. It isn't present on every rhythm strip. The configuration is the most important characteristic of the U wave.

When present, a normal U wave has the following characteristics (amplitude and duration aren't measured):

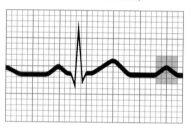

- *location:* follows the T wave
- *configuration:* typically upright and rounded
- *deflection:* upright.

The U wave may not appear on an ECG. A prominent U wave may be due to hypercalcemia, hypokalemia, or digoxin toxicity.

Normal sinus rhythm

Before you can recognize an arrhythmia, you first need to be able to recognize normal sinus rhythm. The term *arrhythmia* literally means an absence of rhythm. The more accurate term dysrhythmia means an abnormality in

Recognizing normal sinus rhythm

Normal sinus rhythm, shown below, represents normal impulse conduction through the heart.

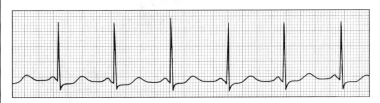

This rhythm strip illustrates normal sinus rhythm.

- *Rhythm:* atrial and ventricular rhythms regular
- *Rate:* atrial and ventricular rates normal, 60 beats/minute
- *P wave:* normal; precedes each QRS complex; all P waves similar in size and shape

- *PR interval:* normal; 0.10 second
- *QRS complex:* 0.06 second
- *T wave:* normal shape (upright and rounded)
- *QT interval:* normal, 0.40 second
- *Other:* no ectopic or aberrantly conducted impulses

rhythm. These terms, however, are frequently used interchangeably.

Normal sinus rhythm records an impulse that starts in the sinus node and progresses to the ventricles through a normal conduction pathway — from the sinus node to the atria and AV node, through the bundle of His, to the bundle branches, and on to the Purkinje fibers. There are no premature or aberrant contractions. Normal sinus rhythm is the standard against which all other rhythms are compared. (See *Recognizing normal sinus rhythm.*)

Practice the eight-step method, described below, to analyze an ECG strip with a normal cardiac rhythm, known as normal sinus rhythm (NSR). The ECG characteristics of NSR include:
■ *rhythm:* atrial and ventricular rhythms are regular

■ *rate:* atrial and ventricular rates 60 to 100 beats/minute, the SA node's normal firing rate
■ *P waves:* normally shaped (round and smooth) and upright in lead II; all P waves similar in size and shape; a P wave for every QRS complex
■ *PR interval:* within normal limits (0.12 to 0.20 second)
■ *QRS complex:* within normal limits (0.06 to 0.10 second)
■ *T wave:* normally shaped; upright and rounded in lead II
■ *QT interval:* within normal limits (0.36 to 0.44 second)
■ *Other:* no ectopic or aberrant beats.

The 8-step method

Analyzing a rhythm strip is a skill developed through practice. You can use several methods, as long as you're consistent. Rhythm strip analysis requires a sequential and systematic approach such as the eight steps outlined here.

STEP 1: DETERMINE RHYTHM

To determine the heart's atrial and ventricular rhythms, use either the paper-and-pencil method or the caliper method. (See *Methods of measuring rhythm.*)

For atrial rhythm, measure the P-P intervals; that is, the intervals between consecutive P waves. These intervals should occur regularly, with only small variations associated with respirations. Then compare the P-P intervals in several cycles. Consistently similar P-P intervals indicate regular atrial rhythm; dissimilar P-P intervals indicate irregular atrial rhythm.

To determine the ventricular rhythm, measure the intervals between two consecutive R waves in the QRS complexes. If an R wave isn't present, use either the Q wave or the S wave of consecutive QRS complexes. The R-R intervals should occur regularly. Then compare R-R intervals in several cycles. As with atrial rhythms, consistently similar intervals mean a regular rhythm; dissimilar intervals point to an irregular rhythm.

After completing your measurements, ask yourself:

■ Is the rhythm regular or irregular? Consider a rhythm with only slight variations, up to 0.04 second, to be regular.

■ If the rhythm is irregular, is it slightly irregular or markedly so? Does the irregularity occur in a pattern (a regularly irregular pattern)?

STEP 2: CALCULATE RATE

You can use one of three methods to determine atrial and ventricular heart rates from an ECG waveform. Although these methods can provide accurate information, you shouldn't rely solely on them when assessing your patient. Keep in mind that the ECG waveform represents electrical, not mechanical, activity. Therefore, although an ECG can show you that ventricular depolarization has occurred, it doesn't mean that ventricular contraction has occurred. To do this, you must assess the patient's pulse. So remember, always check a pulse to correlate it with the heart rate on the ECG.

■ *Times-ten method.* The simplest, quickest, and most common way to calculate rate is the times ten method, especially if the rhythm is irregular. ECG paper is marked in increments of 3 seconds, or 15 large boxes. To calculate the atrial rate, obtain a 6-second strip, count the number of P waves on it, and multiply by 10. Ten 6-second strips equal 1 minute. Calculate ventricular rate the same way, using the R waves.

■ *1,500 method.* If the heart rhythm is regular, use the 1,500 method, so named because 1,500 small squares equals 1 minute. Count the number of small squares between identical points on two consecutive P waves, and then divide 1,500 by that number to get the atrial rate. To obtain the ventricular rate, use the same method with two consecutive R waves.

Methods of measuring rhythm

You can use either of the following methods to determine atrial or ventricular rhythm.

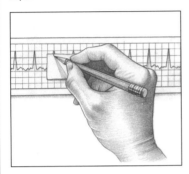

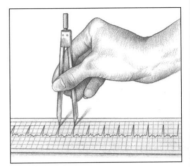

Paper-and-pencil method
Place the ECG strip on a flat surface. Then position the straight edge of a piece of paper along the strip's baseline. Move the paper up slightly so the straight edge is near the peak of the R wave.

With a pencil, mark the paper at the R waves of two consecutive QRS complexes, as shown. This is the R-R interval. Next, move the paper across the strip lining up the two marks with succeeding R-R intervals. If the distance for each R-R interval is the same, the ventricular rhythm is regular. If the distance varies, the rhythm is irregular.

Use the same method to measure the distance between the P waves (the P-P interval) and determine whether the atrial rhythm is regular or irregular.

Caliper method
With the ECG on a flat surface, place one point of the calipers on the peak of the first R wave of two consecutive QRS complexes. Then adjust the caliper legs so the other point is on the peak of the next R wave, as shown. This distance is the R-R interval.

Now pivot the first point of the calipers toward the third R wave and note whether it falls on the peak of that wave. Check succeeding R-R intervals in the same way. If they're all the same, the ventricular rhythm is regular. If they vary, the rhythm is irregular.

Using the same method, measure the P-P intervals to determine whether the atrial rhythm is regular or irregular.

■ *Sequence method.* The third method of estimating heart rate is the sequence method, which requires memorizing a sequence of numbers. For atrial rate, find a P wave that peaks on a heavy black line and assign the following numbers to the next six heavy black lines: 300, 150, 100, 75, 60, and 50. Then find the next P wave peak and estimate the atrial rate, based on the number assigned to the nearest heavy black line. Estimate the ventricular rate the same way, using the R wave.

STEP 3: EVALUATE P WAVE

When examining a rhythm strip for P waves, ask yourself:
- Are P waves present?
- Do the P waves have a normal configuration?
- Do all the P waves have a similar size and shape?
- Is there one P wave for every QRS complex?

STEP 4: DETERMINE PR INTERVAL DURATION

To measure the PR interval, count the small squares between the start of the P wave and the start of the QRS complex; then multiply the number of squares by 0.04 second. After performing this calculation, ask yourself:
- Does the duration of the PR interval fall within normal limits, 0.12 to 0.20 second (or 3 to 5 small squares)?
- Is the PR interval constant?

STEP 5: DETERMINE QRS COMPLEX DURATION

When determining QRS complex duration, make sure you measure straight across from the end of the PR interval to the end of the S wave, not just to the peak. Remember, the QRS complex has no horizontal components. To calculate duration, count the number of small squares between the beginning and end of the QRS complex and multiply this number by 0.04 second. Then ask yourself:
- Does the duration of the QRS complex fall within normal limits, 0.06 to 0.10 second?

- Are all QRS complexes the same size and shape? (If not, measure each one and describe them individually.)
- Does a QRS complex appear after every P wave?

STEP 6: EVALUATE T WAVE

Examine the T waves on the ECG strip. Then ask yourself:
- Are T waves present?
- Do all of the T waves have a normal shape?
- Could a P wave be hidden in a T wave?
- Do all T waves have a normal amplitude?
- Do the T waves have the same the same deflection as the QRS complexes?

STEP 7: DETERMINE QT INTERVAL DURATION

Count the number of small squares between the beginning of the QRS complex and the end of the T wave, where the T wave returns to the baseline. Multiply this number by 0.04 second. Ask yourself:
- Does the duration of the QT interval fall within normal limits, 0.36 to 0.44 second?

STEP 8: EVALUATE OTHER COMPONENTS

Note the presence of ectopic or aberrantly conducted beats or other abnormalities. Also check the ST segment for abnormalities, and look for the presence of a U wave.

Now, interpret your findings by classifying the rhythm strip according to one or all of the following:
- *site of origin of the rhythm:* for example, sinus node, atria, AV node, or ventricles

- *rate:* normal (60 to 100 beats/minute), bradycardia (less than 60 beats/minute), or tachycardia (greater than 100 beats/minute)
- *rhythm:* normal or abnormal; for example, flutter, fibrillation, heart block, escape rhythm, or other arrhythmias.

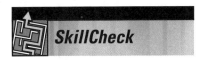

SkillCheck

1. Lead II is one of the:
 a. standard limb leads.
 b. augmented unipolar leads.
 c. modified chest leads.
 d. precordial unipolar leads.
Answer: a. Lead II is one of the standard limb leads, or bipolar limb leads, which have a third electrode known as the ground.

2. The horizontal axis of the ECG strip equals:
 a. 0.1 mV.
 b. 0.04 second.
 c. 0.5 mV.
 d. 0.2 second.
Answer: b. The horizontal axis of the ECG strip represents time. Each small block equals 0.04 second.

3. A monitor problem that appears on the ECG as a thick and unreadable baseline is called:
 a. artifact.
 b. wandering baseline.
 c. electrical interference.
 d. waveform interference.
Answer: c. Electrical interference, or AC interference, is caused by electrical power leakage and appears on the ECG as a baseline that's thick and unreadable.

4. The component of a normal ECG waveform that represents atrial depolarization is the:
 a. P wave.
 b. PR interval.
 c. QRS complex.
 d. T wave.
Answer: a. The P wave is the first component of a normal ECG waveform. It represents atrial depolarization, or conduction of an electrical impulse through the atria.

5. The duration of a normal PR interval is:
 a. 0.5 to 10 mm.
 b. 0.06 to 0.10 second.
 c. 0.12 to 0.20 second.
 d. 0. 36 to 0.44 second.
Answer: c. A normal PR interval has a duration of 0.12 to 0.20 second.

Sinus node arrhythmias

When the heart functions normally, the sinoatrial (SA) node, also called the sinus node, acts as the primary pacemaker. The sinus node assumes this role because its automatic firing rate exceeds that of the heart's other pacemakers. In an adult at rest, the sinus node has an inherent firing rate of 60 to 100 times per minute.

In approximately 50% of the population, the SA node's blood supply comes from the right coronary artery, and from the left circumflex artery in the other half of the population. The autonomic nervous system (ANS) richly innervates the sinus node through the vagal nerve, a parasympathetic nerve, and several sympathetic nerves. Stimulation of the vagus nerve decreases the node's firing rate, and stimulation of the sympathetic system increases it.

Changes in the automaticity of the sinus node, alterations in its blood supply, and ANS influences may all lead to sinus node arrhythmias. This chapter will help you to identify sinus node arrhythmias on an electrocardiogram (ECG). It will also help you to determine the causes, clinical significance, signs and symptoms, and interventions associated with each arrhythmia presented.

The 8-step method to analyze the ECG strip will be used for each of the following arrhythmias.

Sinus arrhythmia

In sinus tachycardia and sinus bradycardia, the cardiac rate falls outside the normal limits. In sinus arrhythmia, the rate stays within normal limits but the rhythm is irregular and corresponds to the respiratory cycle. Sinus arrhythmia can occur normally in athletes, children, and older adults, but it rarely occurs in infants. Conditions unrelated to respiration may also produce sinus arrhythmia, including heart disease, inferior wall myocardial infarction (MI), the use of certain drugs, such as digoxin and morphine, and conditions involving increased intracranial pressure (ICP).

CAUSES

Sinus arrhythmia, the heart's normal response to respirations, results from an inhibition of reflex vagal activity, or tone. During inspiration, an increase in the flow of blood back to the heart reduces vagal tone, which increases the heart rate. ECG complexes fall closer together, which shortens the P-P interval. During expiration, venous return decreases, which in turn increases vagal tone, slows the heart rate, and lengthens the P-P interval. (See *Recognizing sinus arrhythmia.*)

Recognizing sinus arrhythmia

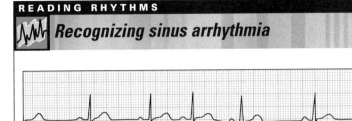

This rhythm strip illustrates sinus arrhythmia.

- *Rhythm:* cyclic, irregular; varies with respiratory cycle
- *Rate:* 60 beats/minute
- *P wave:* normal
- *PR interval:* 0.16 second
- *QRS complex:* 0.06 second
- *T wave:* normal
- *QT interval:* 0.36 second
- *Other:* phasic slowing and quickening

CLINICAL SIGNIFICANCE

Sinus arrhythmia usually isn't significant and produces no symptoms. A marked variation in P-P intervals in an older adult, however, may indicate sick sinus syndrome — a related, potentially more serious phenomenon.

ECG CHARACTERISTICS

■ *Rhythm:* Atrial rhythm is irregular, corresponding to the respiratory cycle. The P-P interval is shorter during inspiration, longer during expiration. The difference between the longest and shortest P-P interval exceeds 0.12 second. Ventricular rhythm is also irregular, corresponding to the respiratory cycle. The R-R interval is shorter during inspiration, longer during expiration. The difference between the longest and shortest R-R interval exceeds 0.12 second.

■ *Rate:* Atrial and ventricular rates are within normal limits (60 to 100 beats/minute) and vary with respiration. Typically, the heart rate increases during inspiration and decreases during expiration.

■ *P wave:* Normal size and configuration; P wave precedes each QRS complex.

■ *PR interval:* May vary slightly within normal limits.

■ *QRS complex:* Normal duration and configuration.

■ *T wave:* Normal size and configuration.

■ *QT interval:* May vary slightly, but usually within normal limits.

■ *Other:* None.

SIGNS AND SYMPTOMS

The patient's peripheral pulse rate increases during inspiration and decreases during expiration. Sinus arrhythmia is easier to detect when the heart rate is slow; it may disappear when the heart rate increases, as with exercise.

If the arrhythmia is caused by an underlying condition, you may note signs and symptoms of that condition. Marked sinus arrhythmia may cause dizziness or syncope in some cases.

INTERVENTIONS
Unless the patient is symptomatic, treatment usually isn't necessary. If sinus arrhythmia is unrelated to respirations, the underlying cause may require treatment.

When caring for a patient with sinus arrhythmia, observe the heart rhythm during respiration to determine whether the arrhythmia coincides with the respiratory cycle. Be sure to check the monitor carefully to avoid an inaccurate interpretation of the waveform.

If sinus arrhythmia is induced by drugs, such as morphine sulfate and other sedatives, the physician may decide to continue to give the patient those medications. If sinus arrhythmia develops suddenly in a patient taking digoxin, notify the physician immediately. The patient may be experiencing digoxin toxicity.

Sinus bradycardia

Sinus bradycardia is characterized by a sinus rate below 60 beats/minute and a regular rhythm. All impulses originate in the SA node. This arrhythmia's significance depends on the symptoms and the underlying cause. Unless the patient shows symptoms of decreased cardiac output, no treatment is necessary. (See *Recognizing sinus bradycardia.*)

CAUSES
Sinus bradycardia usually occurs as the normal response to a reduced demand for blood flow. In this case, vagal stimulation increases and sympathetic stimulation decreases. As a result, automaticity (the tendency of cells to initiate their own impulses) in the SA node diminishes. It may occur normally during sleep or in a person with a well-conditioned heart — an athlete, for instance.

Sinus bradycardia may be caused by:

- noncardiac disorders, such as hyperkalemia, increased ICP, hypothyroidism, hypothermia, and glaucoma
- conditions producing excess vagal stimulation or decreased sympathetic stimulation, such as sleep, deep relaxation, Valsalva's maneuver, carotid sinus massage, and vomiting
- cardiac diseases, such as SA node disease, cardiomyopathy, myocarditis, myocardial ischemia, and heart block; can also occur immediately following an inferior wall MI that involves the right coronary artery, which supplies blood to the SA node.
- certain drugs, especially beta-adrenergic blockers, digoxin, calcium channel blockers, lithium, and antiarrhythmics, such as sotalol, amiodarone, propafenone, and quinidine.

CLINICAL SIGNIFICANCE
The clinical significance of sinus bradycardia depends on how low the rate is and whether the patient is symptomatic. For instance, most adults can tolerate a sinus bradycardia of 45 to 59 beats/minute but are less tolerant of a rate below 45 beats/minute.

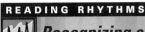

READING RHYTHMS

Recognizing sinus bradycardia

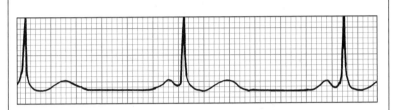

This rhythm strip illustrates sinus bradycardia.

- *Rhythm:* regular
- *Rate:* < 60 beats/minute
- *P wave:* normal; precedes each QRS complex
- *PR interval:* 0.16 second

- *QRS complex:* 0.08 second
- *T wave:* normal
- *QT interval:* 0.50 second
- *Other:* none

Usually, sinus bradycardia is asymptomatic and insignificant. Many athletes develop sinus bradycardia because their well-conditioned hearts can maintain a normal stroke volume with less-than-normal effort. Sinus bradycardia also occurs normally during sleep as a result of circadian variations in heart rate.

When sinus bradycardia is symptomatic, however, prompt attention is critical. The heart of a patient with underlying cardiac disease may not be able to compensate for a drop in rate by increasing its stroke volume. The resulting drop in cardiac output produces such signs and symptoms as hypotension and dizziness. Bradycardia may also predispose some patients to more serious arrhythmias, such as ventricular tachycardia and ventricular fibrillation.

In a patient with acute inferior wall MI, sinus bradycardia is considered a favorable prognostic sign, unless it's accompanied by hypotension. Because sinus bradycardia rarely affects children, it's considered a poor prognostic sign in ill children.

ECG CHARACTERISTICS

■ *Rhythm:* Atrial and ventricular rhythms are regular.

■ *Rate:* Atrial and ventricular rates are less than 60 beats/minute.

■ *P wave:* Normal size and configuration; P wave precedes each QRS complex.

■ *PR interval:* Within normal limits and constant.

■ *QRS complex:* Normal duration and configuration.

■ *T wave:* Normal size and configuration.

■ *QT interval:* Within normal limits, but may be prolonged.

■ *Other:* None.

SIGNS AND SYMPTOMS

The patient will have a pulse rate of less than 60 beats/minute, with a regu-

Bradycardia algorithm

A patient with a bradycardic rhythm may either show few symptoms or show symptoms of decreased cardiac output (CO). If the patient does have decreased CO, determine the cause and initiate appropriate treatments.

Bradycardia
- slow (absolute bradycardia = rate < 60 beats/minute)

  or
- relatively slow (rate less than expected relative to underlying condition or cause)

Primary ABCD survey
- Assess ABCs.
- Secure airway noninvasively.
- Ensure monitor or defibrillator is available.

Secondary ABCD survey
- Assess secondary ABCs (invasive airway management needed?).
- Apply oxygen-I.V. access-monitor-fluids.
- Monitor vital signs, pulse oximeter; monitor blood pressure.
- Obtain and review 12-lead ECG.
- Obtain and review portable chest X-ray.
- Obtain problem-focused history.
- Obtain problem-focused physical examination.
- Consider causes (differential diagnoses).

Serious signs or symptoms?
Due to the bradycardia?

No

Type II second-degree atrioventricular (AV) block or third-degree AV block?

No

Observe.

Yes

- Prepare for transvenous pacer.
- If symptoms develop, use transcutaneous pacemaker until transvenous pacer placed.

Yes

Intervention sequence
- atropine I.V. bolus
- transcutaneous pacing if available
- dopamine I.V. infusion
- epinephrine I.V. infusion

lar rhythm. As long as he's able to compensate for the decreased cardiac output, he's likely to remain asymptomatic. If compensatory mechanisms fail, however, signs and symptoms of declining cardiac output usually appear, including:

- hypotension
- cool, clammy skin
- altered mental status
- dizziness
- blurred vision
- crackles, dyspnea, and an S_3 heart sound, indicating heart failure
- chest pain
- syncope.

Palpitations and pulse irregularities may occur if the patient experiences ectopy such as premature atrial, junctional, or ventricular contractions. This is because the SA node's increased relative refractory period permits ectopic firing. Bradycardia-induced syncope (Stokes-Adams attack) may also occur.

INTERVENTIONS

If the patient is asymptomatic and his vital signs are stable, treatment generally isn't necessary. Continue to observe his heart rhythm, monitoring the progression and duration of the bradycardia. Evaluate his tolerance of the rhythm at rest and with activity. Review the medications he's taking. Check with the physician about stopping medications that may be depressing the SA node, such as digoxin, beta blockers, or calcium channel blockers. Before giving these drugs, make sure the heart rate is within a safe range.

If the patient is symptomatic, treatment aims to identify and correct the underlying cause. Meanwhile, the heart rate must be maintained with such drugs as atropine, dopamine, and epinephrine or with a transvenous or transcutaneous pacemaker. (See *Bradycardia algorithm.*) Keep in mind that a patient with a transplanted heart won't respond to atropine and may require pacing for emergency treatment. Treatment of chronic, symptomatic sinus bradycardia requires insertion of a permanent pacemaker.

Sinus tachycardia

Sinus tachycardia is an acceleration of the firing of the SA node beyond its normal discharge rate. Sinus tachycardia in an adult is characterized by a sinus rate of more than 100 beats/minute. The rate rarely exceeds 180 beats/minute except during strenuous exercise; the maximum rate achievable with exercise decreases with age. (See *Recognizing sinus tachycardia,* page 48.)

CAUSES

Sinus tachycardia may be a normal response to exercise, pain, stress, fever, or strong emotions, such as fear and anxiety. Other causes of sinus tachycardia include:

- certain cardiac conditions, such as heart failure, cardiogenic shock, and pericarditis
- other conditions, such as shock, anemia, respiratory distress, pulmonary embolism, sepsis, and hyperthyroidism where the increased heart rate serves as a compensatory mechanism
- drugs, such as atropine, isoproterenol, aminophylline, dopamine, dobutamine, epinephrine, alcohol, caffeine, nicotine, and amphetamines.

Recognizing sinus tachycardia

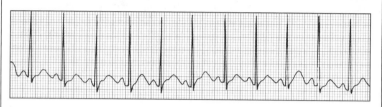

This rhythm strip illustrates sinus tachycardia.

- *Rhythm:* regular
- *Rate:* > 110 beats/minute
- *P wave:* normal; precedes each QRS complex
- *PR interval:* 0.14 second
- *QRS complex:* 0.06 second
- *T wave:* normal
- *QT interval:* 0.34 second
- *Other:* none

CLINICAL SIGNIFICANCE

The clinical significance of sinus tachycardia depends on the underlying cause. The arrhythmia may be the body's response to exercise or high emotional states and of no clinical significance. It may also occur with hypovolemia, hemorrhage, or pain. When the stimulus for the tachycardia is removed, the arrhythmia generally resolves spontaneously.

Although sinus tachycardia commonly occurs without serious adverse effects, persistent sinus tachycardia can also be serious, especially if it occurs in the setting of an acute MI. Tachycardia can lower cardiac output by reducing ventricular filling time and stroke volume. Normally, ventricular volume reaches 120 to 130 ml during diastole. In tachycardia, decreased ventricular volume leads to decreased cardiac output with subsequent hypotension and decreased peripheral perfusion.

Tachycardia worsens myocardial ischemia by increasing the heart's demand for oxygen and reducing the duration of diastole, the period of greatest coronary blood flow. Sinus tachycardia occurs in about 30% of patients after an acute MI and is considered a poor prognostic sign because it may be associated with massive heart damage.

An increase in heart rate can also be detrimental for patients with obstructive types of heart conditions, such as aortic stenosis and hypertrophic cardiomyopathy. Persistent tachycardia may also signal impending heart failure or cardiogenic shock. Sinus tachycardia can also cause angina in patients with coronary artery disease.

ECG CHARACTERISTICS

■ *Rhythm:* Atrial and ventricular rhythms are regular.
■ *Rate:* Atrial and ventricular rates are greater than 100 beats/minute, usually between 100 and 160 beats/minute.

- *P wave:* Normal size and configuration, but it may increase in amplitude. The P wave precedes each QRS complex, but as the heart rate increases, the P wave may be superimposed on the preceding T wave and difficult to identify.
- *PR interval:* Within normal limits and constant.
- *QRS complex:* Normal duration and configuration.
- *T wave:* Normal size and configuration.
- *QT interval:* Within normal limits, but commonly shortened.
- *Other:* None.

SIGNS AND SYMPTOMS

The patient will have a peripheral pulse rate above 100 beats/minute, but with a regular rhythm. Usually, he'll be asymptomatic. However, if his cardiac output falls and compensatory mechanisms fail, he may experience hypotension, syncope, and blurred vision. He may report chest pain and palpitations, often described as a pounding chest or a sensation of skipped heartbeats. He may also report a sense of nervousness or anxiety. If heart failure develops, he may exhibit crackles, an extra heart sound (S_3), and jugular vein distention.

INTERVENTIONS

Treatment usually isn't required unless the patient demonstrates signs and symptoms of decreased cardiac output or hemodynamic instability. The focus of treatment in the symptomatic patient with sinus tachycardia is to maintain adequate cardiac output and tissue perfusion and to identify and correct the underlying cause. For example, if the tachycardia is caused by hemorrhage, treatment includes stopping the bleeding and replacing blood and fluid losses.

If tachycardia leads to cardiac ischemia, treatment may include medications to slow the heart rate. The most commonly used drugs include beta-adrenergic blockers, such as metoprolol and atenolol, and calcium channel blockers such as verapamil.

Check the patient's medication history. Over-the-counter sympathomimetic agents, which mimic the effects of the sympathetic nervous system, may contribute to the sinus tachycardia. Sympathomimetic agents may be contained in nose drops and cold formulas.

Also question the patient about the use of caffeine, nicotine, and alcohol, each of which can trigger tachycardia. Advise him to avoid these substances. Ask about the use of illicit drugs, such as cocaine and amphetamines, which can also cause tachycardia.

Here are other steps you should take for the patient with sinus tachycardia:
- Because sinus tachycardia can lead to injury of the heart muscle, assess the patient for signs and symptoms of angina. Also assess for signs and symptoms of heart failure, including crackles, an S_3 heart sound, and jugular venous distention.
- Monitor intake and output, along with daily weight.
- Check the patient's level of consciousness to assess cerebral perfusion.
- Provide the patient with a calm environment. Help to reduce fear and anxiety, which can aggravate the arrhythmia.
- Teach about procedures and treatments. Include relaxation techniques in the information you provide.

■ Be aware that a sudden onset of sinus tachycardia after an MI may signal extension of the infarction. Prompt recognition is vital so treatment can be started.

■ Keep in mind that tachycardia is frequently the initial sign of pulmonary embolism. Maintain a high index of suspicion, especially if your patient has predisposing risk factors for thrombotic emboli.

Sinus arrest and sinoatrial exit block

Although sinus arrest and SA or sinus exit block are two separate arrhythmias with different etiologies, they're discussed together because distinguishing the two is often difficult. In addition, there's no difference in their clinical significance and treatment.

In sinus arrest, the normal sinus rhythm is interrupted by an occasional, prolonged failure of the SA node to initiate an impulse. Therefore, sinus arrest is caused by episodes of failure in the automaticity or impulse formation of the SA node. The atria aren't stimulated, and an entire PQRST complex is missing from the ECG strip. Except for this missing complex, or pause, the ECG usually remains normal. When one or two impulses aren't formed, it's called a sinus pause; when three or more impulses aren't formed, it's called a sinus arrest. (See *Recognizing sinus arrest.*)

In sinus exit block, the SA node discharges at regular intervals, but some impulses are delayed or blocked from reaching the atria, resulting long sinus

pauses. Blocks result from failure to conduct impulses, whereas sinus arrest results from failure to form impulses in the SA node. Both arrhythmias cause atrial activity to stop. In sinus arrest, the pause often ends with a junctional escape beat. In sinus exit block, the pause occurs for an indefinite period and ends with a sinus rhythm. (See *Recognizing sinoatrial exit block,* page 52.)

CAUSES

Causes of sinus arrest and sinus exit block include:
■ acute infection
■ sick sinus syndrome
■ sinus node disease, such as fibrosis and idiopathic degeneration
■ increased vagal tone, such as with Valsalva's maneuver, carotid sinus massage, and vomiting
■ digoxin, quinidine, procainamide, and salicylate toxicity
■ excessive doses of beta-adrenergic blockers, such as metoprolol and propranolol
■ cardiac disorders, such as coronary artery disease, acute myocarditis, cardiomyopathy, hypertensive heart disease, and acute inferior wall MI.

CLINICAL SIGNIFICANCE

The clinical significance of these two arrhythmias depends on the patient's symptoms. If the pauses are short and infrequent, the patient will most likely be asymptomatic and not require treatment. He may have a normal sinus rhythm for days or weeks between episodes of sinus arrest or sinus exit block, and he may be totally unaware of the arrhythmia. Pauses of 2 to 3 seconds normally occur in healthy adults during sleep, and occasionally in pa-

Recognizing sinus arrest

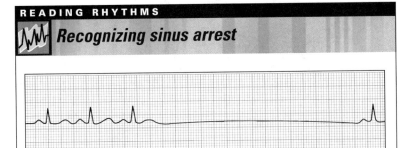

This rhythm strip illustrates sinus arrest.

- *Rhythm:* regular, except for the missing PQRST complexes
- *Rate:* underlying rhythm, 75 beats/minute
- *P wave:* normal; missing during pause
- *PR interval:* 0.20 second

- *QRS complex:* 0.08 second; missing during pause
- *T wave:* normal; missing during pause
- *QT interval:* 0.40 second; missing during pause
- *Other:* none

tients with increased vagal tone or hypersensitive carotid sinus disease.

If either of the arrhythmias is frequent or prolonged, however, the patient will most likely experience symptoms related to low cardiac output. The arrhythmias can produce syncope or near-syncopal episodes usually within 7 seconds of asystole.

During a prolonged pause, the patient may fall and injure himself. Other situations are potentially just as serious. For instance, a symptomatic arrhythmia that occurs while the patient is driving a car could result in a fatal accident. Extremely slow rates can also give rise to other arrhythmias.

ECG CHARACTERISTICS

Both sinus arrest and SA exit block share the following ECG characteristics:

■ *Rhythm:* Atrial and ventricular rhythms are usually regular except for when sinus arrest or SA exit block occurs.

■ *Rate:* The underlying atrial and ventricular rates are usually within normal limits (60 to 100 beats/minute) before the arrest or SA exit block occurs. The length or frequency of the pause may result in bradycardia.

■ *P wave:* Periodically absent, with entire PQRST complex missing. However, when present, the P wave is normal in size and configuration and precedes each QRS complex.

■ *PR interval:* Within normal limits and constant when a P wave is present.

■ *QRS complex:* Normal duration and configuration, but absent during a pause.

■ *T wave:* Normal size and configuration, but absent during a pause.

Recognizing sinoatrial exit block

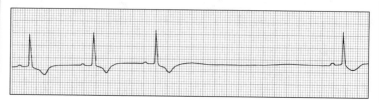

This rhythm strip illustrates sinoatrial (SA) exit block.

- *Rhythm:* regular, except for pauses
- *Rate:* underlying rhythm, 60 beats/ minute) before SA block; length or frequency of the pause may result in bradycardia
- *P wave:* periodically absent
- *PR interval:* 0.16 second
- *QRS complex:* 0.08 second; missing during pause

- *T wave:* normal; missing during pause
- *QT interval:* 0.40 second; missing during pause
- *Other:* entire PQRST complex missing; pause ends with sinus rhythm or atrial escape rhythm

---

- *QT interval:* Usually within normal limits, but absent during a pause.

To differentiate between these two rhythms, compare the length of the pause with the underlying P-P or R-R interval. If the underlying rhythm is regular, determine if the underlying rhythm resumes on time following the pause. With sinus exit block, because the regularity of the SA node discharge is blocked, not interrupted, the underlying rhythm will resume on time following the pause. In addition, the length of the pause will be a multiple of the underlying P-P or R-R interval.

In sinus arrest, the timing of the SA node discharge is interrupted by the failure of the SA node to initiate an impulse. The result is that the underlying rhythm doesn't resume on time after

the pause and the length of the pause is not a multiple of the previous R-R intervals.

SIGNS AND SYMPTOMS

You won't be able to detect a pulse or heart sounds when sinus arrest or sinus exit block occurs. Short pauses usually produce no symptoms, and the patient is asymptomatic. Recurrent or prolonged pauses may cause signs of decreased cardiac output, such as low blood pressure; altered mental status; cool, clammy skin; or syncopal episodes. The patient may also complain of dizziness or blurred vision.

INTERVENTIONS

An asymptomatic patient needs no treatment. Symptomatic patients are treated following the guidelines for patients with symptomatic bradycardia. (See *Bradycardia algorithm,* page 46.) Treatment will also focus on the cause of the sinus arrest or sinus exit block. This may involve discontinuation of medications that contribute to SA node discharge or conduction, such as digoxin, beta blockers, and calcium channel blockers.

Examine the circumstances under which the pauses occur. Both SA arrest and SA exit block may be insignificant if detected while the patient is sleeping. If the pauses are recurrent, assess the patient for evidence of decreased cardiac output, such as altered mental status, low blood pressure, and cool, clammy skin.

Ask him whether he's dizzy or lightheaded or has blurred vision. Does he feel as if he has passed out? If so, he may be experiencing syncope from a prolonged sinus arrest or sinus exit block.

Document the patient's vital signs and how he feels during pauses as well as the activities he was involved in at the time. Activities that increase vagal stimulation, such as Valsalva's maneuver or vomiting, increase the likelihood of sinus pauses.

Assess for a progression of the arrhythmia. Notify the physician immediately if the patient becomes unstable. If appropriate, be alert for signs of digoxin, quinidine, or procainamide toxicity. Obtain a serum digoxin level and a serum electrolyte level.

Sick sinus syndrome

Also known as SA syndrome, sinus nodal dysfunction, and Stokes-Adams syndrome, sick sinus syndrome (SSS) refers to a wide spectrum of SA node arrhythmias. This syndrome is caused by disturbances in the way impulses are generated or in the ability to conduct impulses to the atria. These disturbances may be either intrinsic or mediated by the ANS.

SSS usually shows up as bradycardia, with episodes of sinus arrest and SA block interspersed with sudden, brief periods of rapid atrial fibrillation. Patients are also prone to paroxysms of other atrial tachyarrhythmias, such as atrial flutter and ectopic atrial tachycardia, a condition sometimes referred to as bradycardia-tachycardia (or "brady-tachy") syndrome.

Most patients with SSS are over age 60, but anyone can develop the arrhythmia. It's rare in children except after open-heart surgery that results in SA node damage. The arrhythmia affects men and women equally. The onset is progressive, insidious, and chronic. (See *Recognizing sick sinus syndrome,* page 54.)

CAUSES
SSS results either from a dysfunction of the sinus node's automaticity or from abnormal conduction or blockages of impulses coming out of the nodal region. These conditions, in turn, stem from a degeneration of the area's ANS and partial destruction of the sinus node, as may occur with an interrupted blood supply after an inferior wall MI.

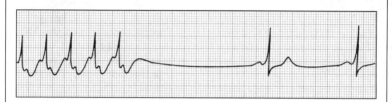

READING RHYTHMS

Recognizing sick sinus syndrome

This rhythm strip illustrates sick sinus syndrome.

- *Rhythm:* irregular
- *Rate:* atrial and ventricular rates fast (150 beats/minute) or slow (43 beats/minute) or alternate between fast and slow; interrupted by a long sinus pause
- *P wave:* varies with prevailing rhythm

- *PR interval:* varies with rhythm
- *QRS complex:* 0.10 second; may vary with rhythm
- *T wave:* configuration varies
- *QT interval:* varies with rhythm changes
- *Other:* sinus pause due to nonfiring sinus node

In addition, certain conditions can affect the atrial wall surrounding the SA node and cause exit blocks. Conditions that cause inflammation or degeneration of atrial tissue can also lead to SSS. In many patients, though, the exact cause is never identified.

Causes of SSS include:
- conditions leading to fibrosis of the SA node, such as increased age, atherosclerotic heart disease, hypertension, and cardiomyopathy
- trauma to the SA node caused by open heart surgery (especially valvular surgery), pericarditis, or rheumatic heart disease
- autonomic disturbances affecting autonomic innervation, such as hypervagotonia or degeneration of the autonomic system

- cardioactive medications, such as digoxin, beta-adrenergic antagonists, and calcium channel blockers.

CLINICAL SIGNIFICANCE

The significance of SSS depends on the patient's age, the presence of other diseases, and the type and duration of the specific arrhythmias that occur. If atrial fibrillation is involved, the prognosis is worse, most likely because of the risk of thromboembolic complications.

If prolonged pauses are involved with SSS, syncope may occur. The length of a pause needed to cause syncope varies with the patient's age, posture at the time, and cerebrovascular status. Any pause that lasts 2 to 3 seconds or more should be considered significant.

A significant part of the diagnosis is whether the patient experiences symptoms while the disturbance occurs. Because the syndrome is progressive and chronic, a symptomatic patient will need lifelong treatment. In addition, thromboembolism may develop as a complication of SSS, possibly resulting in stroke or peripheral embolization.

ECG CHARACTERISTICS

SSS encompasses several potential rhythm disturbances that may be intermittent or chronic. Those rhythm disturbances include one or a combination of the following:

- sinus bradycardia
- SA block
- sinus arrest
- sinus bradycardia alternating with sinus tachycardia
- episodes of atrial tachyarrhythmias, such as atrial fibrillation and atrial flutter
- failure of the sinus node to increase heart rate with exercise.

SSS displays the following ECG characteristics:

- *rhythm:* atrial and ventricular rhythms irregular because of sinus pauses and abrupt rate changes
- *rate:* atrial and ventricular rates fast or slow, or alternate between fast and slow; and interrupted by a long sinus pause
- *P wave:* varies with the prevailing rhythm; may be normal size and configuration or may be absent; when present, a P wave usually precedes each QRS complex
- *PR interval:* usually within normal limits; varies with change in rhythm
- *QRS complex:* duration usually within normal limits; may vary with changes in rhythm; usually normal configuration

- *T wave:* usually normal size and configuration
- *QT interval:* usually within normal limits; varies with rhythm changes
- *Other:* usually more than one arrhythmia on a 6-second strip.

SIGNS AND SYMPTOMS

The patient's pulse rate may be fast, slow, or normal, and the rhythm may be regular or irregular. You can usually detect an irregularity on the monitor or when palpating the pulse, which may feel inappropriately slow, then rapid.

If you monitor the patient's heart rate during exercise or exertion, you may observe an inappropriate response to exercise, such as a failure of the heart rate to increase. You may also detect episodes of brady-tachy syndrome, atrial flutter, atrial fibrillation, SA block, or sinus arrest on the monitor.

Other assessment findings depend on the patient's condition. For instance, he may have crackles in the lungs, S_3, or a dilated and displaced left ventricular apical impulse if he has underlying cardiomyopathy. The patient may also show signs and symptoms of decreased cardiac output, such as fatigue, hypotension, blurred vision, and syncope, a common experience with this arrhythmia. Syncopal episodes, when related to SSS, are referred to as Stokes-Adams attacks.

When caring for a patient with SSS, be alert for signs and symptoms of thromboembolism, especially if the patient has atrial fibrillation. Blood clots or thrombi forming in the heart can dislodge and travel through the bloodstream, resulting in decreased blood supply to the lungs, heart, brain, kidneys, intestines, or other organs. Assess the patient for neurologic changes, such as confusion, vision disturbances, weakness, chest pain, dyspnea, tachypnea, tachycardia, and acute onset of pain. Early recognition allows for prompt treatment.

INTERVENTIONS

As with other sinus node arrhythmias, no treatment is generally necessary if the patient is asymptomatic. If the patient is symptomatic, however, treatment aims to alleviate signs and symptoms and correct the underlying cause of the arrhythmia.

Atropine or epinephrine may be given initially for symptomatic bradycardia. (See *Bradycardia algorithm,* page 46.) A temporary pacemaker may be required until the underlying disorder resolves. Tachyarrhythmias may be treated with antiarrhythmic medications, such as metoprolol and digoxin. Unfortunately, medications used to suppress tachyarrhythmias may worsen underlying SA node disease and bradyarrhythmias.

The patient may need anticoagulants if he develops sudden bursts, or paroxysms, of atrial fibrillation. The anticoagulants help prevent thromboembolism and stroke, a complication of the condition.

When caring for a patient with SSS, monitor and document all arrhythmias as well as signs or symptoms experienced. Note changes in heart rate and rhythm related to changes in the patient's level of activity.

Watch the patient carefully after starting beta blockers, calcium channel blockers, or other antiarrhythmic medications. If treatment includes anticoagulant therapy and pacemaker insertion, make sure the patient and his family receive appropriate instruction.

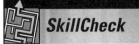

SkillCheck

1. Which of the following is characterized by a rate that stays within normal limits, but a rhythm that's irregular and corresponds to the respiratory cycle?
    a. Sinus arrhythmia
    b. Sinus bradycardia
    c. Sinus tachycardia
    d. Sinus arrest
Answer: a. In sinus arrhythmia, the rate stays within normal limits, but the rhythm is irregular and corresponds to the respiratory cycle.

2. Which of the following worsens myocardial ischemia by increasing the heart's demand for oxygen and reducing the duration of diastole?
    a. Sinus exit block
    b. Sinus arrhythmia
    c. Sinus bradycardia
    d. Sinus tachycardia
Answer: d. Sinus tachycardia worsens myocardial ischemia by increasing the heart's demand for oxygen and reducing the duration of diastole, the period of greatest coronary blood flow.

3. Causes of sinus bradycardia most frequently include:
    a. anemia.
    b. pulmonary embolism.
    c. an inferior wall MI.
    d. hyperthyroidism.
Answer: c. Sinus bradycardia may occur immediately following an inferior wall MI that involves the right coronary artery. The right coronary artery supplies blood to the SA node in 50% of the population.

4. ECG characteristics of SSS include:

    a. regular atrial and ventricular rhythms.

    b. atrial and ventricular rates interrupted by a long sinus pause.

    c. consistently present P waves, which always precede a QRS complex.

    d. consistently prolonged PR intervals.

Answer: b. SSS is characterized by atrial and ventricular rates that are slow or fast, or alternate between slow and fast, and are interrupted by a long sinus pause.

5. Using the 8-step method to analyze the following ECG strip, you would interpret the arrhythmia as:

    a. sinus arrhythmia.

    b. sinus bradycardia.

    c. sinus tachycardia.

    d. sinus arrest.

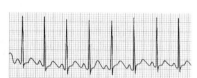

Answer: c. Interpretation: Sinus tachycardia.

Rhythm: Atrial and ventricular rhythms are regular.

Rate: Atrial and ventricular rates are 111 beats per minute.

P wave: Normal size and configuration.

PR interval: 0.14 second.

QRS complex: 0.08 second; normal size and configuration.

T wave: normal configuration.

QT interval: 0.34 second.

Other: None.

Atrial arrhythmias

Atrial arrhythmias, the most common cardiac rhythm disturbances, result from impulses originating in the atrial tissue in areas outside the sinoatrial (SA) node. These arrhythmias can affect ventricular filling time and diminish atrial kick. The term *atrial kick* refers to the complete filling of the ventricles during atrial systole and normally contributes about 25% to ventricular end-diastolic volume.

Atrial arrhythmias are thought to result from three mechanisms: altered automaticity, circus reentry, and afterdepolarization.

■ *Altered automaticity.* The term *automaticity* refers to the ability of cardiac cells to initiate electrical impulses spontaneously. An increase in the automaticity of the atrial fibers can trigger abnormal impulses. Causes of increased automaticity include extracellular factors, such as hypoxia, hypocalcemia, and digoxin toxicity, as well as conditions in which the function of the heart's normal pacemaker, the SA node, is diminished. For example, increased vagal tone or hypokalemia can increase the refractory period of the SA node and allow atrial fibers to initiate impulses.

■ *Circus reentry.* In circus reentry, an impulse is delayed along a slow conduction pathway. Despite the delay, the impulse remains active enough to produce another impulse during myocar-

dial repolarization. Circus reentry may occur with coronary artery disease, cardiomyopathy, or myocardial infarction (MI).

■ *Afterdepolarization.* Afterdepolarization can occur as a result of cell injury, digoxin toxicity, and other conditions. An injured cell sometimes only partially repolarizes. Partial repolarization can lead to repetitive ectopic firing called *triggered activity.* The depolarization produced by triggered activity, known as *afterdepolarization,* can lead to atrial or ventricular tachycardia.

This chapter will help you identify atrial arrhythmias, including premature atrial contractions (PACs), atrial tachycardia, atrial flutter, atrial fibrillation, Ashman's phenomenon, and wandering pacemaker. The chapter reviews causes, clinical significance, electrocardiogram (ECG) characteristics, and signs and symptoms of each arrhythmia as well as interventions directed at treating the patient experiencing these arrhythmias.

Premature atrial contractions

PACs originate in the atria, outside the SA node. They arise from either a single ectopic focus or from multiple atri-

READING RHYTHMS

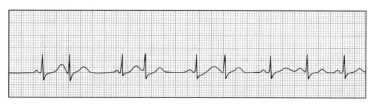

Recognizing premature atrial contractions

This rhythm strip illustrates sinus rhythm with premature atrial contractions (PACs).

- *Rhythm:* irregular
- *Rate:* 90 beats/minute
- *P wave:* premature and abnormally shaped with PACs
- *PR interval:* 0.20 second for the underlying rhythm; unmeasureable for the PAC

- *QRS complex:* 0.08 second
- *T wave:* abnormal with embedded P waves of PACs
- *QT interval:* 0.32 second
- *Other:* noncompensatory pause

al foci that supersede the SA node as pacemaker for one or more beats. PACs are generally caused by enhanced automaticity in the atrial tissue. (See *Recognizing premature atrial contractions.*)

PACs may be conducted or nonconducted (blocked) through the atrioventricular (AV) node and the rest of the heart, depending on the status of the AV and intraventricular conduction system. If the atrial ectopic pacemaker discharges too soon after the preceding QRS complex, the AV junction or bundle branches may still be refractory from conducting the previous electrical impulse. If they're still refractory, they may not be sufficiently repolarized to conduct the premature electrical impulse into the ventricles normally.

When a PAC is conducted, ventricular conduction is usually normal. Nonconducted, or blocked, PACs aren't fol-

lowed by a QRS complex. At times, it may be difficult to distinguish nonconducted PACs from SA block. (See *Distinguishing nonconducted premature atrial contractions from sinoatrial block,* page 60.)

CAUSES

Alcohol, cigarettes, anxiety, fatigue, fever, and infectious diseases can trigger PACs, which commonly occur in a normal heart. Patients who eliminate or control those factors can usually correct the arrhythmia.

PACs may be associated with hyperthyroidism, coronary or valvular heart disease, acute respiratory failure, hypoxia, chronic pulmonary disease, digoxin toxicity, and certain electrolyte imbalances. PACs may also be caused by drugs that prolong the absolute refractory period of the SA node, including quinidine and procainamide.

LOOK-ALIKES

Distinguishing nonconducted premature atrial contractions from sinoatrial block

To differentiate nonconducted premature atrial contractions (PACs) from sinoatrial (SA) block, check the following:

• Whenever you see a pause in a rhythm, look carefully for a nonconducted P wave, which may occur before, during, or just after the T wave preceding the pause.

• Compare T waves that precede a pause with the other T waves in the rhythm strip, looking for a distortion of its slopes or a difference in its height or shape. These are clues showing you where the nonconducted P wave may be hidden.

• If you find a P wave in the pause, check to see whether it's premature or it occurs earlier than subsequent sinus P waves. If it's premature (see shaded area below, top), you can be certain it's a nonconducted PAC.

• If there's no P wave in the pause or T wave (see shaded area below, bottom), then the rhythm is SA block.

Nonconducted PAC

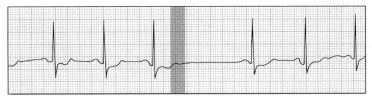

SA block

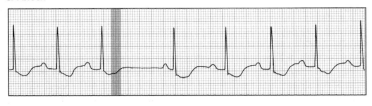

CLINICAL SIGNIFICANCE

PACs are rarely dangerous in patients free of heart disease. They often cause no symptoms and can go unrecognized for years. Patients may perceive PACs as normal palpitations or skipped beats.

However, in patients with heart disease, PACs may lead to more serious arrhythmias, such as atrial fibrillation or atrial flutter. In a patient with acute MI, PACs can serve as an early sign of heart failure or electrolyte imbalance. PACs can also result from endogenous catecholamine release during episodes of pain or anxiety.

ECG CHARACTERISTICS

Rhythm: Atrial and ventricular rhythms are irregular as a result of PACs, but the underlying rhythm may be regular.

Rate: Atrial and ventricular rates vary with the underlying rhythm.

P wave: The hallmark characteristic of a PAC is a premature P wave with an abnormal configuration, when compared with a sinus P wave. Varying configurations of the P wave indicate more than one ectopic site. PACs may be hidden in the preceding T wave.

PR interval: Usually within normal limits but may be either shortened or slightly prolonged for the ectopic beat, depending on the origin of the ectopic focus.

QRS complex: Duration and configuration are usually normal when the PAC is conducted. If no QRS complex follows the PAC, the beat is called a *nonconducted PAC.*

T wave: Usually normal; however, if the P wave is hidden in the T wave, the T wave may appear distorted.

QT interval: Usually within normal limits.

Other: PACs may occur as a single beat, in a bigeminal (every other beat is premature), trigeminal (every third beat), or quadrigeminal (every fourth beat) pattern, or in couplets (pairs). Three or more PACs in a row is called *atrial tachycardia.*

PACs are commonly followed by a pause as the SA node resets. The PAC depolarizes the SA node early, causing it to reset itself and disrupting the normal cycle. The next sinus beat occurs sooner than it normally would, causing a P-P interval between normal beats interrupted by a PAC to be shorter than three consecutive sinus beats, an occurrence referred to as *noncompensatory.*

SIGNS AND SYMPTOMS

The patient may have an irregular peripheral or apical pulse rhythm when the PACs occur. Otherwise, the pulse rhythm and rate will reflect the underlying rhythm. Patients may complain of palpitations, skipped beats, or a fluttering sensation. In a patient with heart disease, signs and symptoms of decreased cardiac output, such as hypotension and syncope, may occur.

INTERVENTIONS

Most asymptomatic patients don't need treatment. If the patient is symptomatic, however, treatment may focus on eliminating the cause, such as caffeine and alcohol. People with frequent PACs may be treated with drugs that prolong the refractory period of the atria. Those drugs include digoxin, procainamide, and propranolol.

When caring for a patient with PACs, assess him to help determine factors that trigger ectopic beats. Tailor patient teaching to help the patient correct or avoid underlying causes. For example, the patient might need to avoid caffeine or learn stress reduction techniques to lessen anxiety.

If the patient has ischemic or valvular heart disease, monitor for signs and symptoms of heart failure, electrolyte imbalance, and more severe atrial arrhythmias.

Atrial tachycardia

Atrial tachycardia is a supraventricular tachycardia, which means that the impulses driving the rapid rhythm originate above the ventricles. Atrial tachycardia has an atrial rate from 150 to

Recognizing atrial tachycardia

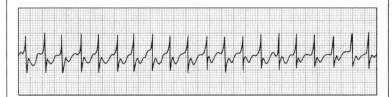

This rhythm strip illustrates atrial tachycardia.

- *Rhythm:* regular
- *Rate:* 210 beats/minute
- *P wave:* hidden in the preceding T wave
- *PR interval:* not visible

- *QRS complex:* 0.10 second
- *T wave:* inverted
- *QT interval:* 0.20 second
- *Other:* T-wave changes (inversion may indicate ischemia)

250 beats/minute. The rapid rate shortens diastole, resulting in a loss of atrial kick, reduced cardiac output, reduced coronary perfusion, and the potential for myocardial ischemia. (See *Recognizing atrial tachycardia.*)

Three forms of atrial tachycardia are discussed here: atrial tachycardia with block, multifocal atrial tachycardia (MAT or chaotic atrial rhythm), and paroxysmal atrial tachycardia (PAT). In MAT, the tachycardia originates from multiple foci. PAT is generally a transient event in which the tachycardia appears and disappears suddenly.

CAUSES

Atrial tachycardia can occur in patients with a normal heart. In those cases, it's commonly related to excessive use of caffeine or other stimulants, marijuana use, electrolyte imbalance, hypoxia, or physical or psychological stress. Typically, however, atrial tachycardia is as-

sociated with primary or secondary cardiac disorders, including MI, cardiomyopathy, congenital anomalies, Wolff-Parkinson-White (WPW) syndrome, and valvular heart disease.

This rhythm may be a component of sick sinus syndrome. Other problems resulting in atrial tachycardia include cor pulmonale, hyperthyroidism, systemic hypertension, and digoxin toxicity, the most common cause of atrial tachycardia.

CLINICAL SIGNIFICANCE

In a healthy person, nonsustained atrial tachycardia is usually benign. However, this rhythm may be a forerunner of more serious ventricular arrhythmias, especially if it occurs in a patient with underlying heart disease.

The increased ventricular rate that occurs in atrial tachycardia results in decreased ventricular filling time, increased myocardial oxygen consumption, and decreased oxygen supply to

Identifying types of atrial tachycardia

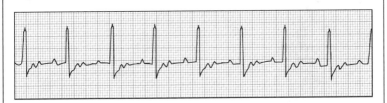

Characteristics of atrial tachycardia with block:

- *Rhythm:* atrial—regular; ventricular—regular if block is constant; irregular if block is variable
- *Rate:* atrial—140 to 250 beats/ minute and a multiple of ventricular rate; ventricular—varies with block
- *P wave:* slightly abnormal

- *PR interval:* can vary but is usually constant for conducted P waves
- *QRS complex:* usually normal
- *T wave:* usually indistinguishable
- *QT interval:* may be indiscernible
- *Other:* more than one P wave for each QRS

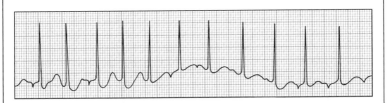

Characteristics of multifocal atrial tachycardia:

- *Rhythm:* both irregular
- *Rate:* atrial—100 to 250 beats/ minute; usually under 160; ventricular—100 to 250 beats/minute
- *P wave:* configuration varying; usu- ally at least three different P-wave shapes must appear

- *PR interval:* varies
- *QRS complex:* usually normal, may become aberrant if arrhythmia per- sists
- *T wave:* usually distorted
- *QT interval:* may be indiscernible
- *Other:* none

(continued)

the myocardium. Heart failure, myo- cardial ischemia, and MI can result.

ECG CHARACTERISTICS

Rhythm: The atrial rhythm is usually regular. The ventricular rhythm is regu- lar or irregular, depending on the AV conduction ratio and the type of atrial tachycardia. (See *Identifying types of atrial tachycardia.*)

Rate: The atrial rate is characterized by three or more consecutive ectopic atrial

Identifying types of atrial tachycardia *(continued)*

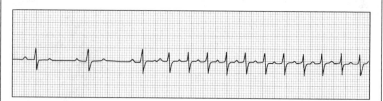

Characteristics of paroxysmal atrial tachycardia:

- *Rhythm:* atrial and ventricular rhythms may be regular or irregular and start and stop abruptly.
- *Rate:* 140 to 250 beats/minute
- *P wave:* may be inverted or retrograde; may not be visible or may be difficult to distinguish from the preceding T wave
- *PR interval:* may be unmeasurable if the P wave can't be distinguished

from the preceding T wave
- *QRS complex:* can be aberrantly conducted
- *T wave:* usually indistinguishable
- *QT interval:* may be indistinguishable
- *Other:* sudden onset, typically initiated by a premature atrial contraction

beats occurring at a rate between 150 and 250 beats/minute. The rate rarely exceeds 250 beats/minute. The ventricular rate depends on the AV conduction ratio.

P wave: The P wave may be aberrant (deviating from normal appearance) or hidden in the preceding T wave. If visible, it's usually upright and precedes each QRS complex.

PR interval: The PR interval may be unmeasurable if the P wave can't be distinguished from the preceding T wave.

QRS complex: Duration and configuration are usually normal, unless the impulses are being conducted abnormally through the ventricles.

T wave: Usually distinguishable but may be distorted by the P wave; may be inverted if ischemia is present.
QT interval: Usually within normal limits but may be shorter because of the rapid rate.
Other: Sometimes it may be difficult to distinguish atrial tachycardia with block from sinus arrhythmia with U waves. (See *Distinguishing atrial tachycardia with block from sinus arrhythmia with U waves.*)

SIGNS AND SYMPTOMS
The patient with atrial tachycardia will have a rapid apical and peripheral pulse rate. The rhythm may be regular or irregular, depending on the type of atrial tachycardia. A patient with PAT may complain that his heart suddenly starts

Distinguishing atrial tachycardia with block from sinus arrhythmia with U waves

Atrial tachycardia with block may appear strikingly similar to sinus arrhythmia with U waves. Always check "normal" rhythm strips carefully to make sure you haven't overlooked or misinterpreted something abnormal. Here's how to tell the difference between the two rhythms.

Atrial tachycardia with block
• Examine the T wave and the interval from the T wave to the next P wave for evidence of extra P waves (see shaded areas below). If you find extra P waves, map them to determine whether they occur at regular intervals with the "normal" P waves.
• In atrial tachycardia with block, the P-P intervals are constant.

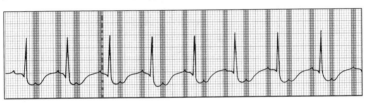

Sinus arrhythmia with U waves
• It's possible to mistake a U wave (see shaded areas below) for an extra P wave. The key is to determine if all of the waves occur at regular intervals. In sinus arrhythmia with U waves, the interval from a U wave to a P wave and a P wave to a U wave won't be constant.

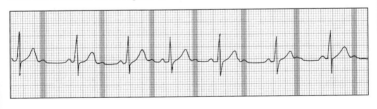

to beat faster or that he suddenly feels palpitations. Persistent tachycardia and rapid ventricular rate cause decreased cardiac output, resulting in hypotension and syncope.

INTERVENTIONS
Treatment depends on the type of tachycardia and the severity of the pa-

tient's symptoms. (See *Tachycardia algorithm,* pages 66 and 67.) Because one of the most common causes of atrial tachycardia is digoxin toxicity, assess the patient for signs and symptoms of digoxin toxicity and monitor digoxin blood levels.

(Text continues on page 68.)

Tachycardia algorithm

The algorithm for tachycardia is complex. Remember to base actions on the type of tachycardia the patient is experiencing and on how the patient is tolerating the rhythm.

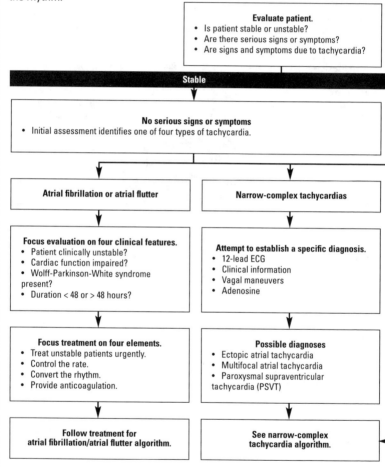

Evaluate patient.
- Is patient stable or unstable?
- Are there serious signs or symptoms?
- Are signs and symptoms due to tachycardia?

Stable

No serious signs or symptoms
- Initial assessment identifies one of four types of tachycardia.

Atrial fibrillation or atrial flutter

Narrow-complex tachycardias

Focus evaluation on four clinical features.
- Patient clinically unstable?
- Cardiac function impaired?
- Wolff-Parkinson-White syndrome present?
- Duration < 48 or > 48 hours?

Attempt to establish a specific diagnosis.
- 12-lead ECG
- Clinical information
- Vagal maneuvers
- Adenosine

Focus treatment on four elements.
- Treat unstable patients urgently.
- Control the rate.
- Convert the rhythm.
- Provide anticoagulation.

Possible diagnoses
- Ectopic atrial tachycardia
- Multifocal atrial tachycardia
- Paroxysmal supraventricular tachycardia (PSVT)

Follow treatment for atrial fibrillation/atrial flutter algorithm.

See narrow-complex tachycardia algorithm.

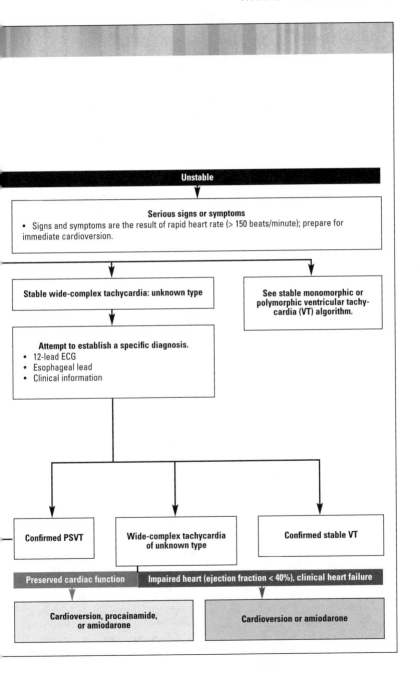

Unstable

Serious signs or symptoms
- Signs and symptoms are the result of rapid heart rate (> 150 beats/minute); prepare for immediate cardioversion.

Stable wide-complex tachycardia: unknown type

See stable monomorphic or polymorphic ventricular tachy-cardia (VT) algorithm.

Attempt to establish a specific diagnosis.
- 12-lead ECG
- Esophageal lead
- Clinical information

Confirmed PSVT

Wide-complex tachycardia of unknown type

Confirmed stable VT

Preserved cardiac function **Impaired heart (ejection fraction < 40%), clinical heart failure**

Cardioversion, procainamide, or amiodarone

Cardioversion or amiodarone

Understanding carotid sinus massage

Carotid sinus massage may be used to interrupt paroxysmal atrial tachycardia. Massaging the carotid sinus stimulates the vagus nerve, which inhibits firing of the sinoatrial (SA) node and slows atrioventricular (AV) node conduction. As a result, the SA node can resume its function as primary pacemaker.

Carotid sinus massage involves a firm massage that lasts no longer than 5 to 10 seconds. The patient's head is turned to the left to massage the right carotid sinus, as demonstrated below. Remember to never attempt simultaneous, bilateral massage.

Carotid sinus massage is contraindicated in patients with carotid bruits. Risks of the procedure include decreased heart rate, syncope, sinus arrest, increased degree of AV block, cerebral emboli, cerebrovascular accident, and asystole.

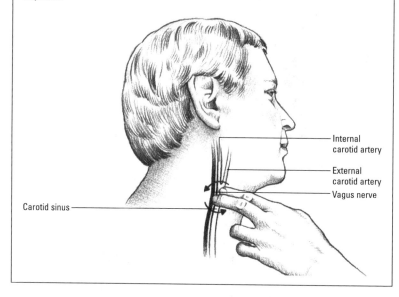

Internal carotid artery

External carotid artery

Vagus nerve

Carotid sinus

The Valsalva maneuver or carotid sinus massage may be used to treat PAT. (See *Understanding carotid sinus massage.*) These maneuvers increase the parasympathetic tone, which results in a slowing of the heart rate. They also allow the SA node to resume function as the primary pacemaker.

Keep in mind that vagal stimulation can result in bradycardia, ventricular arrhythmias, and asystole. (See *Narrow-complex tachycardia algorithm,* page 70.) If vagal maneuvers are used, make sure resuscitative equipment is readily available.

Drug therapy (pharmacologic cardioversion) may be used to increase the degree of AV block and decrease ventricular response rate. Appropriate drugs include digoxin, beta-adrenergic

Narrow-complex tachycardia algorithm

Types of narrow-complex tachycardia include junctional tachycardia, paroxysmal supraventricular tachycardia (PSVT), and multifocal atrial tachycardia (MAT). Treatment for each type of rhythm depends on how well the patient tolerates the rhythm.

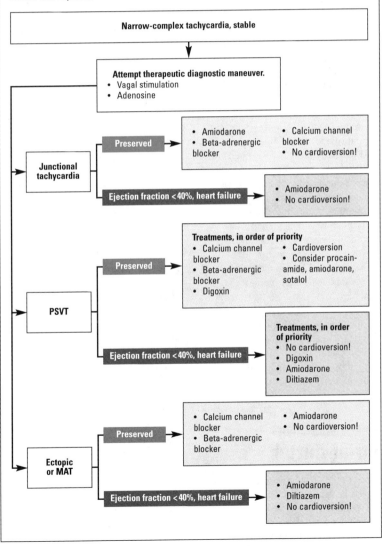

Narrow-complex tachycardia, stable

Attempt therapeutic diagnostic maneuver.
- Vagal stimulation
- Adenosine

Junctional tachycardia

Preserved
- Amiodarone
- Beta-adrenergic blocker
- Calcium channel blocker
- No cardioversion!

Ejection fraction < 40%, heart failure
- Amiodarone
- No cardioversion!

PSVT

Preserved

Treatments, in order of priority
- Calcium channel blocker
- Beta-adrenergic blocker
- Digoxin
- Cardioversion
- Consider procainamide, amiodarone, sotalol

Ejection fraction < 40%, heart failure

Treatments, in order of priority
- No cardioversion!
- Digoxin
- Amiodarone
- Diltiazem

Ectopic or MAT

Preserved
- Calcium channel blocker
- Beta-adrenergic blocker
- Amiodarone
- No cardioversion!

Ejection fraction < 40%, heart failure
- Amiodarone
- Diltiazem
- No cardioversion!

blockers, and calcium channel blockers. When other treatments fail, or if the patient is clinically unstable, synchronized electrical cardioversion may be used.

Atrial overdrive pacing (also called *rapid atrial pacing* or *overdrive suppression*) may also be used to stop the arrhythmia. This technique involves suppression of spontaneous depolarization of the ectopic pacemaker by a series of paced electrical impulses at a rate slightly higher than the intrinsic ectopic atrial rate. The pacemaker cells are depolarized prematurely and, following termination of the paced electrical impulses, the SA node resumes its normal role as the pacemaker.

If the arrhythmia is associated with WPW syndrome, catheter ablation (permanent damage of the area causing the arrhythmia) may be used to control recurrent episodes of PAT. Because MAT often occurs in patients with chronic pulmonary disease, the rhythm may not respond to treatment.

When caring for a patient with atrial tachycardia, carefully monitor the patient's rhythm strips. Doing so may provide information about the cause of atrial tachycardia, which in turn can facilitate treatment. Monitor the patient for chest pain, indications of decreased cardiac output, and signs and symptoms of heart failure or myocardial ischemia.

Atrial flutter

Atrial flutter, a supraventricular tachycardia, is characterized by a rapid atrial rate of 250 to 400 beats/minute, although it's generally around 300 beats/minute. Originating in a single atrial

focus, this rhythm results from circus reentry and possibly increased automaticity.

On an ECG, the P waves lose their normal appearance due to the rapid atrial rate. The waves blend together in a sawtooth configuration called *flutter waves*, or *F waves*. These waves are the hallmark of atrial flutter. (See *Recognizing atrial flutter*.)

CAUSES

Atrial flutter may be caused by conditions that enlarge atrial tissue and elevate atrial pressures. The arrhythmia is often found in patients with mitral or tricuspid valvular disease, hyperthyroidism, pericardial disease, digoxin toxicity, or primary myocardial disease. The rhythm is sometimes encountered in patients following cardiac surgery or in patients with acute MI, chronic pulmonary disease, or systemic arterial hypoxia. Atrial flutter rarely occurs in healthy people. When it does, it may indicate intrinsic cardiac disease.

CLINICAL SIGNIFICANCE

The clinical significance of atrial flutter is determined by the number of impulses conducted through the AV node. That number is expressed as a conduction ratio, such as 2:1 or 4:1, and the resulting ventricular rate. If the ventricular rate is too slow (below 40 beats/minute) or too fast (above 150 beats/minute), cardiac output can be seriously compromised.

Usually the faster the ventricular rate, the more dangerous the arrhythmia. Rapid ventricular rates reduce ventricular filling time and coronary perfusion, which can cause angina, heart failure, pulmonary edema, hypotension, and syncope.

Recognizing atrial flutter

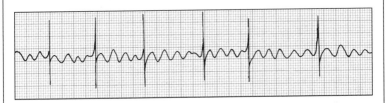

This rhythm strip illustrates atrial flutter.

- *Rhythm:* atrial—regular; ventricular—typically irregular
- *Rate:* atrial—280 beats/minute; ventricular— 60 beats/minute; ventricular rate depends on degree of atrioventricular block
- *P wave:* classic sawtooth appearance referred to as flutter or F waves

- *PR interval:* unmeasurable
- *QRS complex:* 0.08 second; duration usually normal
- *T wave:* unidentifiable
- *QT interval:* unmeasurable
- *Other:* atrial rate—greater than the ventricular rate

ECG CHARACTERISTICS

Rhythm: Atrial rhythm is regular. Ventricular rhythm depends on the AV conduction pattern; it's often regular, although cycles may alternate. An irregular pattern may signal atrial fibrillation or indicate development of a block.

Rate: Atrial rate is 250 to 400 beats/minute. Ventricular rate depends on the degree of AV block; usually it's 60 to 100 beats/minute, but it may accelerate to 125 to 150 beats/minute.

Varying degrees of AV block produce ventricular rates that are usually one-half to one-fourth of the atrial rate. These are expressed as ratios, for example, 2:1 or 4:1. Usually, the AV node won't accept more than 180 impulses/minute and allows every second, third, or fourth impulse to be conducted. These impulses account for the ventricular rate. At the time atrial flutter is initially recognized, the ventricular response is typically above 100 beats/minute. One of the most common ventricular rates is 150 beats/minute with an atrial rate of 300, known as *2:1 block.*

P wave: Atrial flutter is characterized by abnormal P waves that produce a sawtooth appearance, referred to as flutter or F waves.

PR interval: Unmeasurable.

QRS complex: Duration is usually within normal limits, but the complex may be widened if flutter waves are buried within the complex.

T wave: Not identifiable.

QT interval: Unmeasurable because the T wave isn't identifiable.

Other: The patient may develop an atrial rhythm that commonly varies between a fibrillatory line and flutter

Distinguishing atrial flutter from atrial fibrillation

It isn't uncommon to see atrial flutter that has an irregular pattern of impulse conduction to the ventricles. In some leads, this may be confused with atrial fibrillation. Here's how to tell the two arrhythmias apart.

Atrial flutter

• Look for characteristic abnormal P waves that produce a sawtooth appearance, referred to as *flutter waves,* or *F waves.* These can best be identified in leads I, II, and V_1.

• Remember that the atrial rhythm is regular. You should be able to map the F waves across the rhythm strip. While some F waves may occur within the QRS or T waves, subsequent F waves will be visible and occur on time.

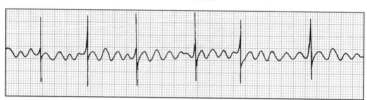

Atrial fibrillation

• Fibrillatory or f waves occur in an irregular pattern, making the atrial rhythm irregular.

• If you identify atrial activity that at times looks like flutter waves and seems to be regular for a short time,

and in other places the rhythm strip contains fibrillatory waves, interpret the rhythm as atrial fibrillation. Coarse fibrillatory waves may intermittently look similar to the characteristic sawtooth appearance of flutter waves.

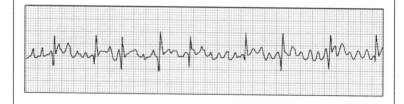

waves. This variation is referred to as atrial fib-flutter. The ventricular response is irregular. At times it may be difficult to distinguish atrial flutter from atrial fibrillation. (See *Distin-*

guishing atrial flutter from atrial fibrillation.)

SIGNS AND SYMPTOMS

When caring for a patient with atrial flutter, you may note that the peripheral and apical pulses are normal in rate and rhythm. That's because the pulse reflects the number of ventricular contractions, not the number of atrial impulses.

If the ventricular rate is normal, the patient may be asymptomatic. If the ventricular rate is rapid, however, the patient may experience a feeling of palpitations and may exhibit signs and symptoms of reduced cardiac output.

INTERVENTIONS

If the patient is hemodynamically unstable, synchronized electrical cardioversion or countershock should be administered immediately. Cardioversion delivers electrical current to the heart to correct an arrhythmia, but unlike defibrillation, it usually uses much lower energy levels and is synchronized to discharge at the peak of the R wave. This causes immediate depolarization, interrupting reentry circuits and allowing the SA node to resume control as pacemaker. Synchronizing the energy current delivery with the R wave ensures that the current won't be delivered on the vulnerable T wave, which could initiate ventricular tachycardia or ventricular fibrillation.

The focus of treatment for hemodynamically stable patients with atrial flutter includes controlling the rate and converting the rhythm. Specific interventions depend on the patient's cardiac function, whether preexcitation syndromes are involved, and the duration (less than or greater than 48 hours) of the arrhythmia. For example, in atrial flutter with normal cardiac function and duration of rhythm less than 48 hours, direct current (DC) cardioversion may be considered; for duration greater than 48 hours, *no DC cardio-version* because it increases the risk of thromboembolism unless the patient has been adequately anticoagulated.

Because atrial flutter may be an indication of intrinsic cardiac disease, monitor the patient closely for signs and symptoms of low cardiac output. Be alert to the effects of digoxin, which depresses the SA node.

If electrical cardioversion is indicated, prepare the patient for I.V. administration of a sedative or anesthetic as ordered. Keep resuscitative equipment at the bedside. Be alert for bradycardia because cardioversion can decrease the heart rate.

Atrial fibrillation

Atrial fibrillation, sometimes called *AFib,* is defined as chaotic, asynchronous, electrical activity in atrial tissue. It results from the firing of multiple impulses from numerous ectopic pacemakers in the atria. Atrial fibrillation is characterized by the absence of P waves and an irregularly irregular ventricular response.

When a number of ectopic sites in the atria initiate impulses, depolarization can't spread in an organized manner. Small sections of the atria are depolarized individually, resulting in the atrial muscle quivering instead of contracting. On an ECG, uneven baseline fibrillatory waves, or f waves, appear rather than clearly distinguishable P waves.

The AV node protects the ventricles from the 400 to 600 erratic atrial impulses that occur each minute by acting as a filter and blocking some of the impulses. The ventricles respond only to

READING RHYTHMS

Recognizing atrial fibrillation

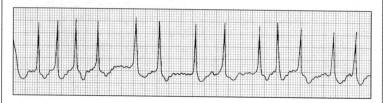

This rhythm strip illustrates atrial fibrillation.

- *Rhythm:* irregularly irregular
- *Rate:* atrial—indiscernible; ventricular—130 beats/minute
- *P wave:* absent; replaced by fine fibrillatory waves, or f waves
- *PR interval:* indiscernible

- *QRS complex:* 0.08 second; duration and configuration are usually normal
- *T wave:* indiscernible
- *QT interval:* unmeasurable
- *Other:* none

impulses conducted through the AV node, hence the characteristic, wide variation in R-R intervals. When the ventricular response rate drops below 100, atrial fibrillation is considered controlled. When the ventricular rate exceeds 100, the rhythm is considered uncontrolled. Atrial fibrillation is considered fast or uncontrolled at rates greater than 100. A "normal" ventricular response is defined as 60 to 100 beats/minute, so a ventricular rate of 100 is considered within normal.

Like atrial flutter, atrial fibrillation results in a loss of atrial kick. The rhythm may be sustained or paroxysmal, meaning that it occurs suddenly and ends abruptly. It can either be preceded by or be the result of PACs. (See *Recognizing atrial fibrillation.*)

CAUSES

Atrial fibrillation occurs more commonly than atrial flutter or atrial tachy-cardia. Atrial fibrillation can occur following cardiac surgery. Other causes of atrial fibrillation include rheumatic heart disease, valvular heart disease (especially mitral valve disease), hyperthyroidism, pericarditis, coronary artery disease, acute MI, hypertension, cardiomyopathy, atrial septal defects, and chronic pulmonary disease.

The rhythm may also occur in a healthy person who smokes or drinks coffee or alcohol or who is fatigued and under stress. Certain drugs, such as aminophylline and digoxin, may contribute to the development of atrial fibrillation. Endogenous catecholamine released during exercise may also trigger the arrhythmia.

CLINICAL SIGNIFICANCE

The loss of atrial kick from atrial fibrillation can result in the subsequent loss of approximately 20% of normal end-diastolic volume. Combined with the decreased diastolic filling time associated with a rapid heart rate, clinically significant reductions in cardiac output can result. In uncontrolled atrial fibrillation, the patient may develop heart failure, myocardial ischemia, or syncope.

Patients with preexisting cardiac disease, such as hypertrophic cardiomyopathy, mitral stenosis, rheumatic heart disease, or those with mitral prosthetic valves, tend to tolerate atrial fibrillation poorly and may develop severe heart failure.

Left untreated, atrial fibrillation can lead to cardiovascular collapse, thrombus formation, and systemic arterial or pulmonary embolism. (See *Risk of restoring sinus rhythm.*)

ECG CHARACTERISTICS

Rhythm: Atrial and ventricular rhythms are grossly irregular, typically described as irregularly irregular.
Rate: The atrial rate is almost indiscernible and usually exceeds 400 beats/minute. The atrial rate far exceeds the ventricular rate because most impulses aren't conducted through the AV junction. The ventricular rate usually varies from 100 to 150 beats/minute but can be below 100 beats/minute.
P wave: The P wave is absent. Erratic baseline f waves appear in place of P waves. These chaotic waves represent atrial tetanization from rapid atrial depolarizations.
PR interval: Indiscernible.
QRS complex: Duration and configuration are usually normal.
T wave: Indiscernible.
QT interval: Unmeasurable.
Other: The patient may develop an atrial rhythm that frequently varies between a fibrillatory line and flutter

> ## *Risk of restoring sinus rhythm*
>
> A patient with atrial fibrillation is at increased risk for developing atrial thrombus and subsequent systemic arterial embolism. In atrial fibrillation, neither atrium contracts as a whole. As a result, blood may pool on the atrial wall, and thrombi may form. Thrombus formation places the patient at higher risk for emboli and stroke.
>
> If normal sinus rhythm is restored and the atria contract normally, clots may break away from the atrial wall and travel through the pulmonary or systemic circulation with potentially disastrous results, such as cerebrovascular accident, pulmonary embolism, or arterial occlusion.

waves, a phenomenon called *atrial fibflutter.* At times it may be difficult to distinguish atrial fibrillation from multifocal atrial tachycardia and from junctional rhythm. (See *Distinguishing atrial fibrillation from multifocal atrial tachycardia,* page 76, and *Distinguishing atrial fibrillation from junctional rhythm,* page 77.)

SIGNS AND SYMPTOMS

When caring for a patient with atrial fibrillation, you may find that the radial pulse rate is slower than the apical rate. The weaker contractions that occur in atrial fibrillation don't produce a palpable peripheral pulse; only the stronger ones do.

The pulse rhythm will be irregularly irregular, with a normal or abnormal heart rate. Patients with a new onset of atrial fibrillation and a rapid ventricular

Distinguishing atrial fibrillation from multifocal atrial tachycardia

To help you decide whether a rhythm is atrial fibrillation, or the similar multifocal atrial tachycardia (MAT), focus on the presence of P waves as well as the atrial and ventricular rhythms. You may find it helpful to look at a longer (greater than 6 seconds) rhythm strip.

Atrial fibrillation
• Carefully look for discernible P waves before each QRS complex.
• If you can't clearly identify P waves, and fibrillatory waves, or f waves, appear in the place of P waves, then the rhythm is probably atrial fibrillation.

• Carefully look at the rhythm, focusing on the R-R intervals. Remember that one of the hallmarks of atrial fibrillation is an irregularly irregular rhythm.

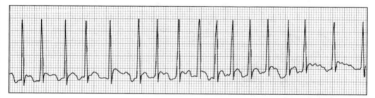

MAT
• P waves are present in MAT. Keep in mind, though, that the shape of the P waves will vary, with at least three different P wave shapes visible in a single rhythm strip.

• You should be able to see most, if not all, the various P wave shapes repeat.
• Although the atrial and ventricular rhythms are irregular, the irregularity generally isn't as pronounced as in atrial fibrillation.

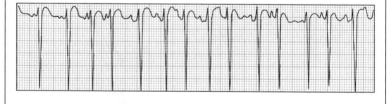

rate may demonstrate signs and symptoms of decreased cardiac output, including hypotension and light-headedness. Patients with chronic atrial fibrillation may be able to compensate for the decreased cardiac output. Although these patients may be asymptomatic, they face a greater-than-normal risk of the development of pulmonary, cerebral, or other thromboembolic events.

LOOK-ALIKES

Distinguishing atrial fibrillation from junctional rhythm

At times, it can be easy to mistake atrial fibrillation for junctional rhythm. Here's how to tell the two apart.

Atrial fibrillation

• Examine lead II, which provides a clear view of atrial activity. Look for fibrillatory waves, or f waves, which appear as a wavy line. These waves indicate atrial fibrillation.

• Chronic atrial fibrillation tends to have fine or small f waves and a controlled ventricular rate (below 100 beats/minute).

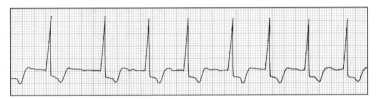

Junctional rhythm

• In lead II, if you can find inverted P waves after or within 0.12 second before the QRS complex (see shaded area below), the rhythm is junctional.
• Assess the patient's jugular veins. Look at the a waves, the normally dominant positive waves in the jugular venous waveform. If cannon a waves are seen with each beat, the rhythm is most likely junctional. Cannon a waves are large a waves indicating that the right atrium is contracting against an increased resistance. Large a waves can occur during arrhythmias whenever the right atrium contracts while the tricuspid valve is closed by right ventricular systole. Regularly occurring cannon waves may be seen during junctional rhythm, whereas a waves are absent in patients with atrial fibrillation.

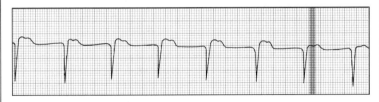

INTERVENTIONS

Treatment of atrial fibrillation aims to reduce the ventricular response rate to below 100 beats/minute. This may be accomplished either by drugs that control the ventricular response or by a combination of electrical cardioversion and drug therapy, to convert the arrhythmia to normal sinus rhythm. When the onset of atrial fibrillation is

How synchronized cardioversion works

A patient experiencing an arrhythmia that leads to reduced cardiac output may be a candidate for synchronized cardioversion. This procedure may be done electively or as an emergency. For instance, it may be used electively in a patient with recurrent atrial fibrillation or urgently in a patient with ventricular tachycardia and a pulse.

Synchronized cardioversion is similar to defibrillation, also called *unsynchronized cardioversion,* except that synchronized cardioversion generally requires lower energy levels. Synchronizing the energy delivered to the patient reduces the risk that the current will strike during the relative refractory period of a cardiac cycle and induce ventricular fibrillation (VF).

In synchronized cardioversion, the R wave on the patient's ECG is synchronized with the cardioverter (defibrillator). Once the firing buttons have been pressed, the cardioverter discharges energy when it senses the next R wave.

Keep in mind that a slight delay occurs between the time the discharge buttons are depressed and the moment the energy is actually discharged. When using handheld paddles, continue to hold the paddles on the patient's chest until the energy is delivered.

Remember to reset the "sync mode" on the defibrillator after each synchronized cardioversion. Resetting this switch is necessary because most defibrillators will automatically reset to an unsynchronized mode.

If VF occurs during the procedure, turn off the sync button and immediately deliver an unsynchronized defibrillation to terminate the arrhythmia. Be aware that synchronized cardioversion carries the risk of lethal arrhythmia when used in patients with digoxin toxicity.

---

acute and the patient can cooperate, vagal maneuvers or carotid sinus massage may slow the ventricular response but won't convert the arrhythmia.

If the patient is hemodynamically unstable, synchronized electrical cardioversion should be administered immediately. Electrical cardioversion is most successful if used within the first 48 hours after onset and less successful the longer the duration of the arrhythmia. Conversion to normal sinus rhythm will cause forceful atrial contractions to resume abruptly. If a thrombus forms in the atria, the resumption of contractions can result in systemic emboli. (See *How synchronized cardioversion works.*)

The focus of treatment for hemodynamically stable patients with atrial fibrillation includes controlling the rate, converting the rhythm, and providing anticoagulation if indicated. Specific interventions depend on the patient's cardiac function, whether preexcitation syndromes are involved, and the duration of the arrhythmia.

Drugs such as digoxin, procainamide, propranolol, quinidine, amiodarone, and verapamil may be given after successful cardioversion to maintain normal sinus rhythm and to control the ventricular rate in chronic atrial fibrillation. Some of these drugs prolong the atrial refractory period, giving the SA node an opportunity to reestablish its role as the heart's pacemaker. Others primarily slow AV node conduction, controlling the ventricular response rate. Symptomatic atrial fibrillation that doesn't respond to routine treatment may be treated with radiofrequency ablation therapy.

When assessing a patient with atrial fibrillation, assess the peripheral and apical pulses. If the patient isn't on a cardiac monitor, be alert for an irregular pulse and differences in the radial and apical pulse rates.

Assess for symptoms of decreased cardiac output and heart failure. If drug therapy is used, monitor serum drug levels and observe the patient for evidence of toxicity. Tell the patient to report pulse rate changes, syncope or dizziness, chest pain, and signs of heart failure, such as dyspnea and peripheral edema.

Ashman's phenomenon

Ashman's phenomenon refers to the aberrant conduction of premature supraventricular beats to the ventricles. (See *Ashman's phenomenon,* page 80.) This benign phenomenon is frequently associated with atrial fibrillation but can occur with any arrhythmia that affects the R-R interval.

CAUSES
Ashman's phenomenon is caused by a prolonged refractory period associated with slower rhythms. In theory, a con-

duction aberration occurs when a short cycle follows a long cycle because the refractory period varies with the length of the cycle. An impulse that ends a short cycle preceded by a long one is more likely to reach refractory tissue.

The normal refractory period for the right bundle branch is slightly longer than the left one, so premature beats frequently reach the right bundle when it's partially or completely refractory. Because of this tendency, the abnormal beat is usually seen as a right bundle branch block (RBBB).

CLINICAL SIGNIFICANCE
The importance of recognizing aberrantly conducted beats is primarily to prevent misdiagnosis and subsequent mistaken treatment of ventricular ectopy.

ECG CHARACTERISTICS
Rhythm: Atrial and ventricular rhythms are irregular.
Rate: Atrial and ventricular rates reflect the underlying rhythm.
P wave: The P wave has an abnormal configuration. It may be visible. If present in the underlying rhythm, the P wave is unchanged.
PR interval: If measurable, the interval often changes on the premature beat.
QRS complex: Configuration is usually altered, revealing an RBBB pattern.
T wave: Deflection opposite that of the QRS complex occurs in most leads as a result of RBBB.
QT interval: Usually has changed as a result of the RBBB.
Other: There's no compensatory pause after an aberrant beat. The aberrancy may continue for several beats and typically ends a short cycle preceded by a long cycle.

READING RHYTHMS

Ashman's phenomenon

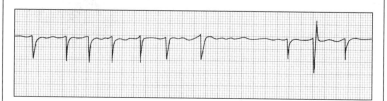

This rhythm strip illustrates Ashman's phenomenon.

- *Rhythm:* atrial and ventricular—irregular
- *Rate:* underlying rhythm of 90 beats/minute
- *P wave:* absent; fibrillatory waves
- *PR interval:* if measurable, the interval commonly changes on the premature beat.
- *QRS complex:* 0.12 second; right bundle-branch block (RBBB) pattern present on Ashman beat

- *T wave:* deflection opposite that of QRS complex in the Ashman beat
- *QT interval:* usually changed due to RBBB
- *Other:* no compensatory pause after the aberrant beat; aberrancy may continue for several beats

SIGNS AND SYMPTOMS
None

INTERVENTIONS
None

Wandering pacemaker

Wandering pacemaker, also called *wandering atrial pacemaker,* is an atrial arrhythmia that results when the site of impulse formation shifts from the SA node to another area above the ventricles. The origin of the impulse may wander beat to beat from the SA node to ectopic sites in the atria, or to the AV junctional tissue. The P wave and PR interval vary from beat to beat as the pacemaker site changes. (See *Recognizing wandering pacemaker.*)

CAUSES
In most cases, wandering pacemaker is caused by increased parasympathetic (vagal) influences on the SA node or AV junction. It can also be caused by chronic pulmonary disease, valvular heart disease, digoxin toxicity, and inflammation of the atrial tissue.

CLINICAL SIGNIFICANCE
The arrhythmia may be normal in young patients and is common in athletes who have slow heart rates. The ar-

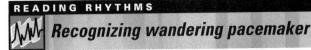

READING RHYTHMS

Recognizing wandering pacemaker

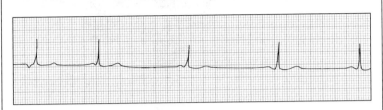

This rhythm strip illustrates wandering pacemaker.

- *Rhythm:* atrial and ventricular—irregular
- *Rate:* atrial and ventricular—50 beats/minute
- *P wave:* changes in size and shape; first P wave inverted, second upright
- *PR interval:* varied
- *QRS complex:* 0.08 second
- *T wave:* normal
- *QT interval:* 0.44 second
- *Other:* none

rhythmia may be difficult to identify because it's often transient. Although wandering pacemaker is rarely serious, chronic arrhythmias are a sign of heart disease and should be monitored.

ECG CHARACTERISTICS

Rhythm: The atrial rhythm varies slightly, with an irregular P-P interval. The ventricular rhythm varies slightly, with an irregular R-R interval.

Rate: Atrial and ventricular rates vary but are usually within normal limits, or below 60 beats/minute.

P wave: Altered size and configuration are due to the changing pacemaker site. The P wave may also be absent, inverted, or may follow the QRS complex if the impulse originates in the AV junction. A combination of these variations may appear.

PR interval: The PR interval varies from beat to beat as the pacemaker site

changes but usually less than 0.20 second. If the impulse originates in the AV junction, the PR interval will be less than 0.12 second. This variation in PR interval will cause a slightly irregular R-R interval. When the P wave is present, the PR interval may be normal or shortened.

QRS complex: Ventricular depolarization is normal, so duration of the QRS complex is usually within normal limits and is of normal configuration.

T wave: Normal size and configuration.

QT interval: Usually within normal limits, but may vary.

Other: At times it may be difficult to distinguish wandering pacemaker from premature atrial contractions. (See *Distinguishing wandering pacemaker from premature atrial contractions.*)

Distinguishing wandering pacemaker from premature atrial contractions

Because premature atrial contractions (PACs) are commonly encountered, it's possible to mistake wandering pacemaker for PACs unless the rhythm strip is carefully examined. In such cases, you may find it helpful to look at a longer (greater than 6 seconds) rhythm strip.

Wandering pacemaker
• Carefully examine the P waves. You must be able to identify at least three different shapes of P waves (see shaded areas below) in wandering pacemaker.

• Atrial rhythm varies slightly, with an irregular P-P interval. Ventricular rhythm varies slightly, with an irregular R-R interval. These slight variations in rhythm result from the changing site of impulse formation.

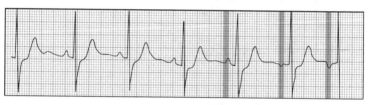

PAC
• The PAC occurs earlier than the sinus P wave, with an abnormal configuration when compared with a sinus P wave (see shaded area below). It's possible, but rare, to see multifocal PACs, which originate from multi-

ple ectopic pacemaker sites in the atria. In this setting, the P waves may have different shapes.
• With the exception of the irregular atrial and ventricular rhythms as a result of the PAC, the underlying rhythm is usually regular.

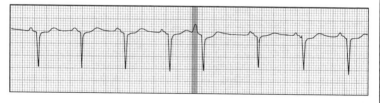

SIGNS AND SYMPTOMS
Patients are generally asymptomatic and unaware of the arrhythmia. The pulse rate may be normal or below 60 beats/minute, and the rhythm may be regular or slightly irregular.

INTERVENTIONS
Usually, no treatment is needed for asymptomatic patients. If the patient is symptomatic, however, the patient's medications should be reviewed and the underlying cause investigated and treated. Monitor the patient's heart

rhythm and assess for signs of hemo-dynamic instability, such as hypotension and changes in mental status.

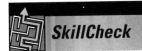
SkillCheck

1. Which of the following events refers to the aberrant conduction of premature supraventricular beats to the ventricle and can occur with any arrhythmia affecting the R-R interval?
   a. Ashman's phenomenon
   b. Atrial tachycardia
   c. Multifocal atrial tachycardia
   d. Wandering pacemaker
Answer: a. Ashman's phenomenon refers to the aberrant or abnormal conduction of premature supraventricular beats to the ventricles. This benign phenomenon is frequently associated with atrial fibrillation but can occur with any arrhythmia that affects the R-R interval.

2. Using the 8-step method of ECG analysis, interpret the following arrhythmia.

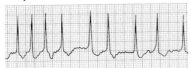

Answer:
Rhythm: Atrial and ventricular rhythms are irregular.
Rate: Atrial rate can't be determined; ventricular rate varies.
P wave: Absent; coarse fibrillatory waves present.
PR interval: Indiscernible.
QRS complex: Normal duration and

configuration.
T wave: Indiscernible.
QT interval: Unmeasurable.
Other: None.
Interpretation: Atrial fibrillation.

3. Using the 8-step method of ECG analysis, interpret the following arrhythmia.

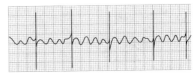

Answer:
Rhythm: Atrial and ventricular rhythms are regular.
Rate: Atrial rate is 250 to 400 beats/minute; ventricular rate varies from 60 to 100 beats/minute.
P wave: Sawtooth pattern; flutter waves.
PR interval: Unmeasurable.
QRS complex: Normal duration.
T wave: Not identifiable.
QT interval: Unmeasurable.
Other: None.
Interpretation: Atrial flutter.

4. Using the 8-step method of ECG analysis, interpret the following arrhythmia.

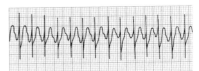

Answer:
Rhythm: Atrial and ventricular rhythms are regular.
Rate: Atrial rate and ventricular rates are 160 to 250 beats/minute.
P wave: Distorted.
PR interval: Unmeasurable; P wave can't be distinguished from the preceding T wave.

QRS complex: Normal duration.
T wave: Indistinguishable.
QT interval: Can't be determined.
Other: None.
Interpretation: Atrial tachycardia.

5. Using the 8-step method of ECG analysis, interpret the following arrhythmia.

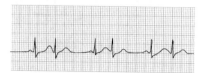

Answer:
Rhythm: Atrial and ventricular rhythms are irregular.
Rate: Atrial and ventricular rates vary.
P wave: Normal size and configuration.
PR interval: Normal for underlying rhythm.
QRS complex: Normal duration and configuration.
T wave: Normal configuration.
QT interval: Within normal limits.
Other: None.
Interpretation: Normal sinus rhythm with premature atrial contractions.

Junctional arrhythmias

Junctional arrhythmias originate in the atrioventricular (AV) junction — the area in and around the AV node and the bundle of His. The specialized pacemaker cells in the AV junction take over as the heart's pacemaker if the sinoatrial (SA) node fails to function properly or if the electrical impulses originating in the SA node are blocked. These junctional pacemaker cells have an inherent firing rate of 40 to 60 beats/minute.

In normal impulse conduction, the AV node slows transmission of the impulse from the atria to the ventricles, which allows the ventricles to fill as much as possible before they contract. However, these impulses don't always follow the normal conduction pathway. (See *Conduction in Wolff-Parkinson-White syndrome,* page 86.)

Because of the location of the AV junction within the conduction pathway, electrical impulses originating in this area cause abnormal depolarization of the heart. The impulse is conducted in a retrograde (backward) fashion to depolarize the atria, and antegrade (forward) to depolarize the ventricles.

Depolarization of the atria can precede depolarization of the ventricles, or the ventricles can be depolarized before the atria. Depolarization of the atria and ventricles can also occur simultaneously. (See *Locating the P wave,* page 87.) Retrograde depolar-

ization of the atria results in inverted P waves in leads II, III, and aV_F, leads in which you would normally see upright P waves appear.

Keep in mind that arrhythmias causing inverted P waves on an electrocardiogram (ECG) may originate in the atria or AV junction. Atrial arrhythmias are sometimes mistaken for junctional arrhythmias because impulses are generated so low in the atria that they cause retrograde depolarization and inverted P waves. Looking at the PR interval will help you determine whether an arrhythmia is atrial or junctional.

An arrhythmia with an inverted P wave before the QRS complex and with a normal PR interval (0.12 to 0.20 second) originates in the atria. An arrhythmia with a PR interval less than 0.12 second originates in the AV junction.

Premature junctional contractions

A premature junctional contraction (PJC) is a junctional beat that occurs before a normal sinus beat and causes an irregular rhythm. These ectopic beats commonly occur as a result of enhanced automaticity in the junctional

Conduction in Wolff-Parkinson-White syndrome

Electrical impulses in the heart don't always follow normal conduction pathways. In preexcitation syndromes, electrical impulses enter the ventricles from the atria through an accessory pathway that bypasses the atrioventricular junction. Wolff-Parkinson-White (WPW) syndrome is a common type of preexcitation syndrome.

WPW syndrome commonly occurs in young children and in adults ages 20 to 35. The syndrome causes the PR interval to shorten and the QRS complex to lengthen as a result of a delta wave. Delta waves, which in WPW occur just before normal ventricular depolarization, are produced as a result of the premature depolarization or preexcitation of a portion of the ventricles.

WPW is clinically significant because the accessory pathway—in this case, Kent's bundle—may result in paroxysmal tachyarrhythmias by reentry and rapid conduction mechanisms.

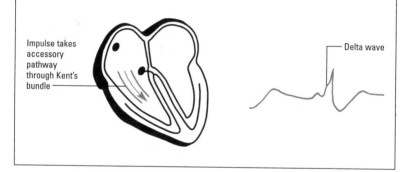

Impulse takes accessory pathway through Kent's bundle

Delta wave

tissue or bundle of His. As with all impulses generated in the AV junction, the atria are depolarized in a retrograde fashion, causing an inverted P wave. The ventricles are depolarized normally. (See *Recognizing a premature junctional contraction,* page 88.)

CAUSES

PJCs may be caused by digoxin toxicity, excessive caffeine intake, amphetamine ingestion, alcohol, stress, coronary artery disease, myocardial ischemia, valvular heart disease, valvular disease, pericarditis, heart failure,

chronic pulmonary disease, hyperthyroidism, electrolyte imbalances, or inflammatory changes in the AV junction following heart surgery.

CLINICAL SIGNIFICANCE

PJCs are generally considered harmless unless they occur frequently—usually defined as more than six per minute. Frequent PJCs indicate junctional irritability and can precipitate a more serious arrhythmia, such as junctional tachycardia. In patients taking digoxin, PJCs are a common early sign of toxicity.

Locating the P wave

When the specialized pacemaker cells in the atrioventricular junction take over as the dominant pacemaker of the heart:
- depolarization of the atria can precede depolarization of the ventricles
- the ventricles can be depolarized before the atria
- simultaneous depolarization of the atria and ventricles can occur.

The rhythm strips shown here demonstrate the various locations of the P waves in junctional arrhythmias, depending on the direction of depolarization.

Inverted P wave
If the atria are depolarized first, the P wave will occur before the QRS complex.

Inverted P wave
If the ventricles are depolarized first, the P wave will occur after the QRS complex.

Inverted P wave (hidden)
If the ventricles and atria are depolarized simultaneously, the P wave will be hidden in the QRS complex.

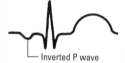

Inverted P wave

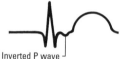

Inverted P wave

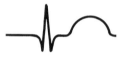

ECG CHARACTERISTICS

Rhythm: Atrial and ventricular rhythms are irregular during PJCs; the underlying rhythm may be regular.
Rate: Atrial and ventricular rates reflect the underlying rhythm.
P wave: The P wave is usually inverted. It may occur before or after the QRS complex, be absent, or be hidden in the QRS complex. Look for an inverted P wave in leads II, III, and aV_F. Depending on the initial direction of depolarization, the P wave may fall before, during, or after the QRS complex.
PR interval: If the P wave precedes the QRS complex, the PR interval is shortened (less than 0.12 second); otherwise, it can't be measured.
QRS complex: Because the ventricles are usually depolarized normally, the QRS complex usually has a normal configuration and a normal duration of less than 0.12 second.
T wave: Usually normal configuration.
QT interval: Usually within normal limits.
Other: A noncompensatory pause reflecting retrograde atrial conduction commonly accompanies PJCs.

SIGNS AND SYMPTOMS

The patient is usually asymptomatic. He may complain of palpitations or a feeling of "skipped heart beats." You may be able to palpate an irregular pulse when PJCs occur. If PJCs are frequent enough, the patient may experience hypotension from a transient decrease in cardiac output.

INTERVENTIONS

PJCs usually don't require treatment unless the patient is symptomatic. In

Recognizing a premature junctional contraction

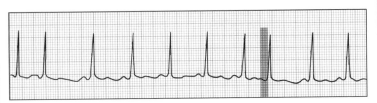

This rhythm strip illustrates sinus rhythm with premature junctional contractions (PJCs).

- *Rhythm:* irregular atrial and ventricular rhythms during PJCs
- *Rate:* 100 beats/minute
- *P wave:* inverted and precedes the QRS complex (see shaded area)
- *PR interval:* 0.14 second for the underlying rhythm and 0.06 second for the PJC

- *QRS complex:* 0.06 second
- *T wave:* normal configuration
- *QT interval:* 0.36 second
- *Other:* noncompensatory pause reflecting retrograde atrial conduction commonly accompanies PJCs

those cases, the underlying cause should be treated. For example, in digoxin toxicity, the medication should be discontinued and serum drug levels monitored.

Monitor the patient for hemodynamic instability as well. If ectopic beats occur frequently, the patient should decrease or eliminate his caffeine intake.

Junctional escape rhythm

A junctional escape rhythm, also referred to as junctional rhythm, is an arrhythmia originating in the AV junction. In this arrhythmia, the AV junc-

tion takes over as a secondary, or "escape" pacemaker. This usually occurs only when a higher pacemaker site in the atria, usually the SA node, fails as the heart's dominant pacemaker.

Remember that the AV junction can take over as the heart's dominant pacemaker if the firing rate of the higher pacemaker sites falls below the AV junction intrinsic firing rate, if the pacemaker fails to generate an impulse, or if the conduction of the impulses is blocked. Because junctional escape beats prevent ventricular standstill, they should never be suppressed.

In a junctional escape rhythm, as in all junctional arrhythmias, the atria are depolarized by means of retrograde conduction. The P waves are inverted, and impulse conduction through the

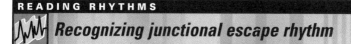

READING RHYTHMS

Recognizing junctional escape rhythm

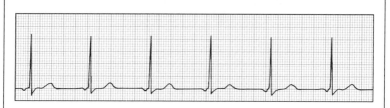

This rhythm strip illustrates junctional escape rhythm.

- *Rhythm:* regular
- *Rate:* 60 beats/minute
- *P wave:* inverted and preceding each QRS complex
- *PR interval:* 0.10 second

- *QRS complex*: 0.10 second
- *T wave:* normal
- *QT interval:* 0.44 second
- *Other:* none

ventricles is normal. The normal intrinsic firing rate for cells in the AV junction is 40 to 60 beats/minute. (See *Recognizing junctional escape rhythm.*)

CAUSES

A junctional escape rhythm can be caused by any condition that disturbs normal SA node function or impulse conduction. Causes of the arrhythmia include SA node ischemia, hypoxia, electrolyte imbalances, valvular heart disease, heart failure, cardiomyopathy, myocarditis, sick sinus syndrome, and increased parasympathetic (vagal) tone. Drugs such as digoxin, calcium channel blockers, and beta-adrenergic blockers can also cause a junctional escape rhythm.

CLINICAL SIGNIFICANCE

The clinical significance of junctional escape rhythm depends on how well the patient tolerates a decreased heart rate (40 to 60 beats/minute) and associated decrease in cardiac output. In addition to a decreased cardiac output from a slower heart rate, depolarization of the atria either after or simultaneously with ventricular depolarization results in loss of atrial kick. Remember that junctional escape rhythms protect the heart from potentially life-threatening ventricular escape rhythms.

ECG CHARACTERISTICS

Rhythm: Atrial and ventricular rhythms are regular.

Rate: The atrial and ventricular rates are 40 to 60 beats/minute.

P wave: The P wave is usually inverted (look for inverted P waves in leads II, III, and aV$_F$). The P wave may occur before or after the QRS complex, be hidden within it, or may be absent.

PR interval: If the P wave precedes the QRS complex, the PR interval is short-

LOOK-ALIKES

Distinguishing atrial fibrillation with third-degree atrioventricular block from junctional rhythm

Although third-degree atrioventricular (AV) block occurs infrequently, it can happen in association with atrial fibrillation. The resulting ventricular rhythm will be regular. If the block occurs at the level of the AV node, a junctional escape pacemaker usually initiates ventricular depolarization. This event results in a normally shaped, narrow QRS complex and a ventricular rate of 40 to 60 beats/minute.

Differentiating the cause of the arrhythmias is key because even though the escape rhythm is a junctional rhythm, patient management of the conditions may differ.

Atrial fibrillation with third-degree AV block
- On lead II, which provides a clear view of atrial activity, search for fibril-latory waves, or f waves, indicating atrial fibrillation.
- Assess the patient's jugular veins. A waves will be absent with atrial fibrillation.

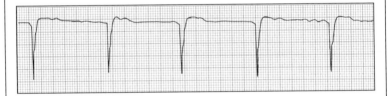

Junctional rhythm
- Inverted P waves either after or within 0.12 second before the QRS complex on lead II indicate junctional rhythm.
- Assess the patient's jugular veins. Large a waves, called cannon a waves, occur with junctional rhythm.

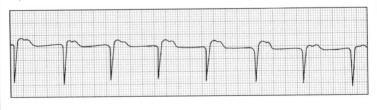

ened (less than 0.12 second); otherwise, it can't be measured.

QRS complex: Duration is usually within normal limits; configuration is usually normal.
T wave: Usually normal configuration.

LOOK-ALIKES

Distinguishing accelerated idioventricular rhythm from junctional rhythm

Idioventricular rhythm and junctional rhythm appear similar but have different causes. To distinguish between the two, closely examine the duration of the QRS complex and then look for P waves.

Accelerated idioventricular rhythm
- The QRS duration will be greater than 0.12 second.
- The QRS will have a wide and bizarre configuration.

- P waves are usually absent.
- The ventricular rate is generally between 40 and 100 beats/minute.

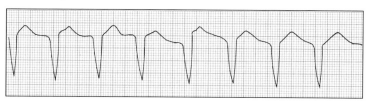

Junctional rhythm
- The QRS duration and configuration are usually normal.
- Inverted P waves generally occur before or after the QRS complex.

However, remember that the P waves may also be absent or buried within the QRS complex.
- The ventricular rate is typically between 40 and 60 beats/minute.

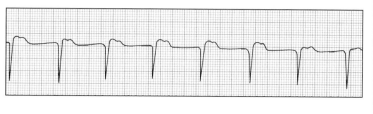

QT interval: Usually within normal limits.
Other: None.
Junctional rhythm can sometimes be difficult to distinguish from atrial fibrillation with third-degree AV block or from an idioventricular rhythm. (See *Distinguishing atrial fibrillation with third-degree atrioventricular block*

from junctional rhythm, and *Distinguishing accelerated idioventricular rhythm from junctional rhythm.*)

SIGNS AND SYMPTOMS

A patient with a junctional escape rhythm will have a slow, regular pulse rate of 40 to 60 beats/minute. The patient may be asymptomatic. However, pulse rates under 60 beats/minute may lead to inadequate cardiac output, causing hypotension, syncope, or blurred vision.

INTERVENTIONS
Treatment for a junctional escape rhythm involves identification and correction of the underlying cause, whenever possible. (See *Bradycardia algorithm,* page 46.) Atropine may be used to increase the heart rate, or a temporary or permanent pacemaker may be inserted.

Monitor the patient's serum digoxin and electrolyte levels and watch for signs of decreased cardiac output, such as hypotension, syncope, and blurred vision.

Accelerated junctional rhythm

An accelerated junctional rhythm is an arrhythmia that originates in the AV junction and is usually caused by enhanced automaticity of the AV junctional tissue. It's called *accelerated* because it occurs at a rate of 60 to 100 beats/minute, exceeding the inherent junctional escape rate of 40 to 60 beats/minute.

Because the rate is below 100 beats/minute, the arrhythmia isn't classified as junctional tachycardia. The atria are depolarized by means of retrograde conduction, and the ventricles are depolarized normally. (See *Recognizing accelerated junctional rhythm.*)

CAUSES
Digoxin toxicity is a common cause of accelerated junctional rhythm. Other causes include electrolyte disturbances, valvular heart disease, rheumatic heart disease, heart failure, myocarditis, cardiac surgery, and inferior- or posterior-wall myocardial infarction.

CLINICAL SIGNIFICANCE
Patients experiencing accelerated junctional rhythm are generally asymptomatic because the rate corresponds to the normal inherent firing rate of the SA node (60 to 100 beats/minute). However, symptoms of decreased cardiac output, including hypotension and syncope, can occur if atrial depolarization occurs after or simultaneously with ventricular depolarization, which causes the subsequent loss of atrial kick.

ECG CHARACTERISTICS
Rhythm: Atrial and ventricular rhythms are regular.
Rate: Atrial and ventricular rates range from 60 to 100 beats/minute.
P wave: If the P wave is present, it will be inverted in leads II, III, and aV$_F$. It may precede, follow, or be hidden in the QRS complex or absent entirely.
PR interval: If the P wave occurs before the QRS complex, the PR interval is shortened (less than 0.12 second). Otherwise, it can't be measured.
QRS complex: Duration is usually within normal limits, though it may be slightly prolonged. Configuration is usually normal.
T wave: Usually within normal limits.
QT interval: Usually within normal limits.
Other: None.

READING RHYTHMS

Recognizing accelerated junctional rhythm

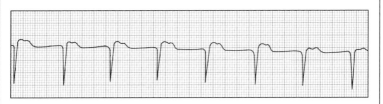

This rhythm strip illustrates accelerated junctional rhythm.

- *Rhythm:* regular
- *Rate:* 80 beats/minute
- *P wave:* absent
- *PR interval:* unmeasurable

- *QRS complex:* 0.10 second
- *T wave:* normal
- *QT interval:* 0.32 second
- *Other:* none

SIGNS AND SYMPTOMS

The pulse rate will be normal with a regular rhythm. The patient may be asymptomatic because accelerated junctional rhythm has the same rate as sinus rhythm. However, if cardiac output is decreased, the patient may exhibit symptoms, such as hypotension, changes in mental status, and weak peripheral pulses.

INTERVENTIONS

Treatment for accelerated junctional rhythm involves identifying and correcting the underlying cause. Assessing the patient for signs and symptoms related to decreased cardiac output and hemodynamic instability is key, as is monitoring serum digoxin and electrolyte levels.

Junctional tachycardia

In junctional tachycardia, three or more premature junctional contractions occur in a row. This supraventricular tachycardia generally occurs as a result of enhanced automaticity of the AV junction, which causes the AV junction to override the SA node as the dominant pacemaker.

In junctional tachycardia, the atria are depolarized by retrograde conduction. Conduction through the ventricles is normal. The rate is usually 100 to 200 beats/minute. (See *Recognizing junctional tachycardia,* page 94.)

CAUSES

Digoxin toxicity is the most common cause of junctional tachycardia. In such cases, the arrhythmia can be aggravated by hypokalemia. Other causes of junc-

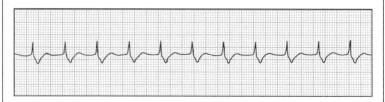

Recognizing junctional tachycardia

This rhythm strip illustrates junctional tachycardia.

- *Rhythm:* atrial and ventricular — regular
- *Rate:* atrial and ventricular — 115 beats/minute
- *P wave:* inverted; follows QRS complex

- *PR interval:* unmeasurable
- *QRS complex:* 0.08 second
- *T wave:* normal
- *QT interval:* 0.36 second
- *Other:* none

---

tional tachycardia include inferior- or posterior-wall infarction or ischemia, inflammation of the AV junction following heart surgery, heart failure, electrolyte imbalances, and valvular heart disease.

CLINICAL SIGNIFICANCE

The clinical significance of junctional tachycardia depends on the rate and underlying cause. At higher ventricular rates, junctional tachycardia may reduce cardiac output by decreasing ventricular filling time. A loss of atrial kick also occurs with atrial depolarization that follows or occurs simultaneously with ventricular depolarization.

ECG CHARACTERISTICS

Rhythm: Atrial and ventricular rhythms are usually regular. The atrial rhythm may be difficult to determine if the

P wave is absent or hidden in the QRS complex or preceding T wave.

Rate: Atrial and ventricular rates exceed 100 beats/minute (usually between 100 and 200 beats/minute). The atrial rate may be difficult to determine if the P wave is absent or hidden in the QRS complex or the preceding T wave.

P wave: The P wave is usually inverted in leads II, III, and aV$_F$. The P wave may occur before or after the QRS complex, be hidden in the QRS complex, or be absent.

PR interval: If the P wave precedes the QRS complex, the PR interval is shortened (less than 0.12 second); otherwise, the PR interval can't be measured.

QRS complex: Duration is within normal limits; configuration is usually normal.

T wave: Configuration is usually normal but may be abnormal if the P wave

is hidden in the T wave. The fast rate may make T waves indiscernible.
QT interval: Usually within normal limits.
Other: None.

SIGNS AND SYMPTOMS

The patient's pulse rate will be above 100 beats/minute and have a regular rhythm. Patients with a rapid heart rate may experience signs and symptoms of decreased cardiac output and hemodynamic instability including hypotension.

INTERVENTIONS

The underlying cause should be identified and treated. If the cause is digoxin toxicity, the drug should be discontinued. Vagal maneuvers and drugs such as verapamil may slow the heart rate for symptomatic patients. Patients with recurrent junctional tachycardia may be treated with ablation therapy, followed by permanent pacemaker insertion.

Monitor patients with junctional tachycardia for signs of decreased cardiac output. In addition, check digoxin and potassium levels and administer potassium supplements as ordered. In some cases of digoxin toxicity, a digoxin-binding drug may be used to reduce serum digoxin levels.

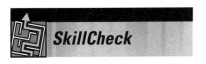

SkillCheck

1. In junctional arrhythmias, the P wave occurs after the QRS complex when the:
   a. ventricles and atria are depolarized spontaneously.

   b. atria are depolarized before the ventricles.
   c. atria aren't depolarized.
   d. ventricles are depolarized before the atria.
Answer: d. Whenever the ventricles are depolarized before the atria, the P wave will be located following the QRS complex.

2. Using the 8-step method of ECG analysis, interpret the following arrhythmia.

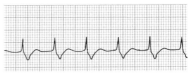

Answer:
Rhythm: Atrial and ventricular rhythms are regular.
Rate: Atrial and ventricular rates are 115 beats/minute.
P wave: Inverted; follows QRS complex.
PR interval: Unmeasurable.
QRS complex: 0.08 second.
T wave: Normal.
QT interval: 0.36 second.
Other: None.
Interpretation: Junctional tachycardia.

3. Using the 8-step method of ECG analysis, interpret the following arrhythmia.

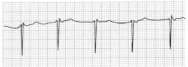

Answer:
Rhythm: Atrial and ventricular rhythms are regular.
Rate: Atrial and ventricular rates are 71 beats/minute.

P wave: Follows QRS complex.
PR interval: Unmeasurable.
QRS complex: 0.08 second; normal size and configuration.
T wave: Normal configuration.
QT interval: 0.36 second.
Other: None.
Interpretation: Accelerated junctional rhythm.

4. Using the 8-step method of ECG analysis, interpret the following arrhythmia.

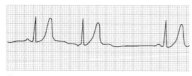

Answer:
Rhythm: Atrial and ventricular rhythms are irregular.
Rate: Atrial and ventricular rates are 40 beats/minute.
P wave: Inverted on second beat.
PR interval: 0.08 second (second beat); 0.16 second (other beats).
QRS complex: 0.08 second.
T wave: Tall and peaked.
QT interval: 0.48 second.
Other: None.
Interpretation: Sinus bradycardia with one premature junctional contraction.

5. Using the 8-step method of ECG analysis, interpret the following arrhythmia.

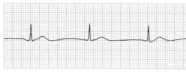

Answer:
Rhythm: Atrial and ventricular rhythms are regular.

Rate: Atrial and ventricular rates are 47 beats/minute.
P wave: Inverted.
PR interval: 0.08 second.
QRS complex: 0.06 second.
T wave: Normal configuration.
QT interval: 0.42 second.
Other: None.
Interpretation: Junctional rhythm.

Ventricular arrhythmias

Ventricular arrhythmias originate in the ventricles below the bifurcation of the bundle of His. These arrhythmias occur when electrical impulses depolarize the myocardium using a different pathway from normal impulse conduction.

Ventricular arrhythmias appear on an electrocardiogram (ECG) in characteristic ways. The QRS complex in most of these arrhythmias is wider than normal because of the prolonged conduction time through, and abnormal depolarization of, the ventricles. The deflections of the T wave and the QRS complex are in opposite directions because ventricular repolarization, as well as ventricular depolarization, is abnormal. The P wave in many ventricular arrhythmias is absent because atrial depolarization doesn't occur.

When electrical impulses come from the ventricles instead of the atria, atrial kick is lost and cardiac output can decrease by as much as 30%. As a result, patients with ventricular arrhythmias may show signs and symptoms of heart failure, including hypotension, angina, syncope, and respiratory distress.

Although ventricular arrhythmias may be benign, they may also be serious because the ventricles are ultimately responsible for cardiac output. Rapid recognition and treatment of ventricular arrhythmias increases the chances of successful resuscitation.

Premature ventricular contractions

Premature ventricular contractions (PVCs) are ectopic beats that originate in the ventricles and occur earlier than expected. PVCs may occur in healthy people without being clinically significant.

However, when PVCs occur in patients with underlying heart disease, they may herald the development of lethal ventricular arrhythmias, including ventricular tachycardia (VT) and ventricular fibrillation (VF).

PVCs may occur singly, in pairs (couplets), or in clusters. PVCs may also appear in patterns, such as bigeminy or trigeminy. (See *Recognizing premature ventricular contractions,* page 98.) In many cases, PVCs are followed by a compensatory pause. PVCs may be uniform in appearance, arising from a single ectopic ventricular pacemaker site, or multiform, originating from a single pacemaker site but having QRS complexes that differ in size, shape, and direction.

PVCs may also be described as unifocal or multifocal. Unifocal PVCs originate from the same ventricular ectopic pacemaker site, whereas multifo-

Recognizing premature ventricular contractions

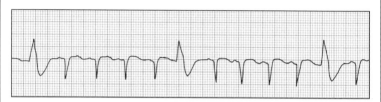

This rhythm strip illustrates normal sinus rhythm with premature ventricular contractions (PVCs).

- *Rhythm:* irregular
- *Rate:* 120 beats/minute
- *P wave:* none with PVC, but P wave present with other QRS complexes
- *PR interval:* 0.12 second in underlying rhythm
- *QRS complex:* early, with bizarre configuration and duration of 0.14

second in PVC; QRS complexes are 0.08 second in underlying rhythm
- *T wave:* normal; opposite direction from QRS complex
- *QT interval:* 0.28 second with underlying rhythm
- *Other:* none

cal PVCs originate from different ectopic pacemaker sites in the ventricles.

CAUSES

PVCs are usually caused by enhanced automaticity in the ventricular conduction system or muscle tissue. The irritable focus results from a disruption of the normal electrolyte shifts during cellular depolarization and repolarization. Possible causes of PVCs include:

- electrolyte imbalances, such as hypokalemia, hyperkalemia, hypomagnesemia, and hypocalcemia
- metabolic acidosis
- hypoxia
- myocardial ischemia and infarction
- drug intoxication, particularly with cocaine, amphetamines, and tricyclic antidepressants

- enlargement or hypertrophy of the ventricular chambers
- increased sympathetic stimulation
- myocarditis
- caffeine or alcohol ingestion
- tobacco use
- irritation of the ventricles by pacemaker electrodes or a pulmonary artery catheter
- sympathomimetic drugs, such as epinephrine and isoproterenol.

CLINICAL SIGNIFICANCE

PVCs are significant for two reasons. First, they can lead to more serious arrhythmias, such as VT or VF. The risk of developing a more serious arrhythmia increases in patients with ischemic or damaged hearts.

PVCs also decrease cardiac output, especially if ectopic beats are frequent or sustained. The decrease in cardiac output with a PVC stems from reduced ventricular diastolic filling time and the loss of atrial kick for that beat. The clinical impact of PVCs hinges on the body's ability to maintain adequate perfusion and the duration of the abnormal rhythm.

To help determine the seriousness of PVCs, ask yourself these questions:

■ *How often do they occur?* In patients with chronic PVCs, an increase in frequency or a change in the pattern of PVCs from the baseline rhythm may signal a more serious condition.

■ *What's the pattern of PVCs?* If the ECG shows a dangerous pattern — such as paired PVCs, PVCs with more than one focus, a bigeminal rhythm, or R-on-T phenomenon (when a PVC strikes on the down slope of the preceding normal T wave) — the patient may require immediate treatment. (See *Patterns of potentially dangerous premature ventricular contractions,* pages 100 and 101.)

■ *Are they really PVCs?* Make sure the complex is a PVC, not another, less dangerous arrhythmia. PVCs may be mistaken for ventricular escape beats or normal impulses with aberrant ventricular conduction. Ventricular escape beats serve as a safety mechanism to protect the heart from ventricular standstill. Some supraventricular impulses may follow an abnormal conduction pathway causing an abnormal appearance to the QRS complex. In any event, never delay treatment if the patient is unstable.

ECG CHARACTERISTICS

Rhythm: Atrial and ventricular rhythms are irregular during PVCs; the underlying rhythm may be regular.

Rate: Atrial and ventricular rates reflect the underlying rhythm.

P wave: Usually absent in the ectopic beat, but with retrograde conduction to the atria, the P wave may appear after the QRS complex. It's usually normal if present in the underlying rhythm.

PR interval: Unmeasurable except in the underlying rhythm.

QRS complex: Occurrence is earlier than expected. Duration exceeds 0.12 second, with a bizarre and wide configuration. Configuration of the QRS complex is usually normal in the underlying rhythm.

T wave: Occurrence is in opposite direction to QRS complex. When a PVC strikes on the down slope of the preceding normal T wave — the R-on-T phenomenon — it can trigger more serious rhythm disturbances.

QT interval: Not usually measured, except in the underlying rhythm.

Other: A PVC may be followed by a compensatory pause, which can be full or incomplete. The sum of a full compensatory pause and the preceding R-R interval is equal to the sum of two R-R intervals of the underlying rhythm. If the sinoatrial (SA) node is depolarized by the PVC, the timing of the SA node is reset, and the compensatory pause is called *incomplete.* In this case, the sum of an incomplete compensatory pause and the preceding R-R interval is less than the sum of two R-R intervals of the underlying rhythm. A PVC occurring between two normally conducted QRS complexes without greatly disturbing the underlying rhythm is referred to as *interpolated.* A full com-

Patterns of potentially dangerous premature ventricular contractions

Some premature ventricular contractions (PVCs) are more dangerous than others. Here are examples of patterns of potentially dangerous PVCs.

Paired PVCs

Two PVCs in a row, called *paired PVCs* or a *ventricular couplet* (see shaded areas), can produce ventricular tachycardia (VT). That's because

the second contraction usually meets refractory tissue. A burst, or a salvo, of three or more PVCs in a row is considered a run of VT.

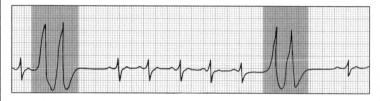

Multiform PVCs

Multiform PVCs, which look different from one another, arise from different sites or from the same site with

abnormal conduction. (See shaded areas.) Multiform PVCs may indicate severe heart disease or digoxin toxicity.

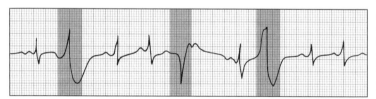

Bigeminy and trigeminy

PVCs that occur every other beat (bigeminy) or every third beat (trigeminy) can result in VT or ven-

tricular fibrillation. (See shaded areas.) The rhythm strip shown below illustrates ventricular bigeminy.

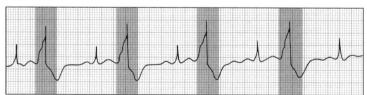

Patterns of potentially dangerous premature ventricular contractions (continued)

R-on-T phenomenon
In R-on-T phenomenon, a PVC occurs so early that it falls on the T wave of the preceding beat (See shaded area.) Because the cells haven't fully repolarized, VT or VF can result.

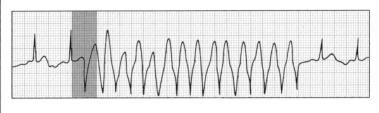

pensatory pause, usually accompanying PVCs, is absent with interpolated PVCs.

Sometimes it's difficult to distinguish PVCs from aberrant ventricular conduction. (See *Distinguishing premature ventricular contractions from ventricular aberrancy,* pages 102 and 103.)

SIGNS AND SYMPTOMS

A patient with PVCs usually has a pulse rate within the normal range of 60 to 100 beats/minute. When a PVC occurs, the pulse rhythm will be momentarily irregular.

With PVCs, the patient will have a weaker pulse wave after the premature beat and a longer-than-normal pause between pulse waves. At times, you may not be able to palpate a pulse after the PVC. If the carotid pulse is visible, however, you may see a weaker arterial wave after the premature beat. When auscultating for heart sounds, you'll hear an abnormally early heart sound with each PVC.

A patient with PVCs may be asymptomatic. However, patients with frequent PVCs may complain of palpitations. The patient may also exhibit signs and symptoms of decreased cardiac output, including hypotension and syncope.

INTERVENTIONS

If the patient is asymptomatic and doesn't have heart disease, the arrhythmia probably won't require treatment. If symptoms or a dangerous form of PVCs occur, the type of treatment given will depend on the cause of the problem.

If PVCs have a purely cardiac origin, drugs to suppress ventricular irritability may be used. Procainamide, amiodarone, and lidocaine are typically used. When PVCs have a noncardiac origin, treatment is aimed at correcting the cause. For example, drug therapy may be adjusted or the patient's acidosis corrected.

Patients who have recently developed PVCs need prompt assessment,

Distinguishing premature ventricular contractions from ventricular aberrancy

Perhaps one of the most challenging look-alikes—premature ventricular contractions (PVCs) versus ventricular aberrancy—can sometimes be distinguished with complete confidence only in the electrophysiology laboratory. Ventricular aberrancy, or aberrant ventricular conduction, occurs when an electrical impulse originating in the sinoatrial node, atria, or atrioventricular junction is temporarily conducted abnormally through the bundle branches.

The abnormal conduction results in a bundle-branch block and usually stems from the arrival of electrical impulses at the bundle branches before the branches have been sufficiently repolarized.

To distinguish between PVCs and ventricular aberrancy, examine the deflection of the QRS complex in lead V_1. Determine whether the QRS complex is primarily positive or negative. Based on this information, follow these clues to guide your analysis.

Mostly positive QRS
• Right bundle-branch aberrancy will have a triphasic rSR' configuration in V_1 and a triphasic qRS configuration in V_6.

• If there are two positive peaks in V_1 and the left peak is taller, the beat is probably a PVC.
• PVCs will be monophasic or biphasic in V_1, and biphasic in V_6, with a deep S wave.

Comparing PVC with right bundle-branch aberrancy

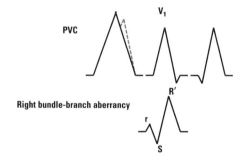
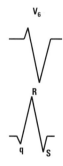

(continued)

especially if they have underlying heart disease or complex medical problems. Patients with chronic PVCs should be observed closely for the development

of more frequent PVCs or more dangerous PVC patterns.

Until effective treatment is begun, patients with PVCs accompanied by serious symptoms should have continu-

Distinguishing premature ventricular contractions from ventricular aberrancy *(continued)*

Mostly negative QRS
• Left bundle-branch aberrancy will have a narrow R wave with a quick downstroke in leads V_1 and V_2, and no Q wave in V_6.
• PVCs will have a wide R wave (> 0.03 second) and a notched or slurred S-wave downstroke in leads V_1 and V_2, with a duration of > 0.06 second from the onset of the R wave

to the deepest point of the S wave in V_1 and V_2, and a Q wave in V_6.
• P waves commonly precede aberrancies. P waves don't generally precede PVCs.
• Aberrancies usually have a QRS duration of 0.12 second. PVCs are more likely to have a QRS duration of 0.14 second or more.

Comparing PVC with left bundle-branch aberrancy

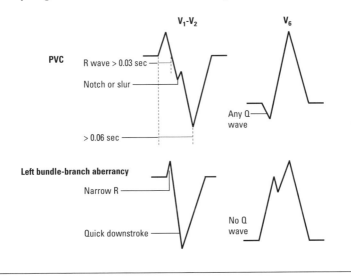

ous ECG monitoring and ambulate only with assistance. If the patient is discharged on antiarrhythmic medications, family members should know how to contact the emergency medical system and perform cardiopulmonary resuscitation (CPR).

Idioventricular rhythm

Idioventricular rhythm, also referred to as *ventricular escape rhythm,* originates in an escape pacemaker site in the ventricles. The inherent firing rate

Recognizing idioventricular rhythm

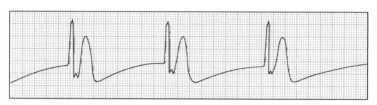

This rhythm strip illustrates idioventricular rhythm.

- *Rhythm:* irregular
- *Rate:* atrial — unable to determine; ventricular — 30 beats/minute
- *P wave:* absent
- *PR interval:* unmeasurable

- *QRS complex:* 0.20 second; wide and bizarre
- *T wave:* directly opposite last part of QRS complex
- *QT interval:* 0.46 second
- *Other:* none

of this ectopic pacemaker is usually 30 to 40 beats/minute. The rhythm acts as a safety mechanism by preventing ventricular standstill, or asystole — the absence of electrical activity in the ventricles. When fewer than three QRS complexes arising from the escape pacemaker occur, they're called *ventricular escape beats* or *complexes.* (See *Recognizing idioventricular rhythm.*)

When the rate of an ectopic pacemaker site in the ventricles is under 100 beats/minute but exceeds the inherent ventricular escape rate of 30 to 40 beats/minute, it's called *accelerated idioventricular rhythm* or *AIVR.* (See *Recognizing accelerated idioventricular rhythm.*) The rate of AIVR isn't fast enough to be considered VT. The rhythm is usually related to enhanced automaticity of the ventricular tissue. AIVR and idioventricular rhythm share the same ECG characteristics, differing only in heart rate.

CAUSES

Idioventricular rhythms occur when all of the heart's higher pacemakers fail to function or when supraventricular impulses can't reach the ventricles because of a block in the conduction system. Idioventricular rhythms may accompany third-degree heart block. Possible causes of the rhythm include:
- myocardial ischemia
- myocardial infarction (MI)
- digoxin toxicity, beta-adrenergic blockers, calcium antagonists, and tricyclic antidepressants
- pacemaker failure
- metabolic imbalances.

CLINICAL SIGNIFICANCE

Idioventricular rhythm may be transient or continuous. Transient ventricular escape rhythm is usually related to

WARNING

Recognizing accelerated idioventricular rhythm

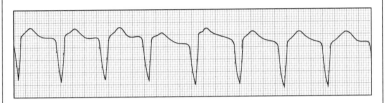

This rhythm strip illustrates accelerated idioventricular rhythm.

- *Rhythm:* regular
- *Rate:* ventricular — 80 beats/minute
- *P wave:* absent; sometimes inverted P wave follows the QRS complex
- *PR interval:* unmeasurable

- *QRS complex:* 0.18 second; wide and bizarre
- *T wave:* 0.48 second
- *QT interval:* usually prolonged
- *Other:* none

increased parasympathetic effect on the higher pacemaker sites and isn't generally clinically significant. Although idioventricular rhythms act to protect the heart from ventricular standstill, a continuous idioventricular rhythm presents a clinically serious situation.

The slow ventricular rate of this arrhythmia and the associated loss of atrial kick markedly reduce cardiac output. If not rapidly identified and appropriately managed, idioventricular arrhythmias can cause death.

ECG CHARACTERISTICS

Rhythm: Usually, atrial rhythm can't be determined. Ventricular rhythm is usually regular.
Rate: Usually, atrial rate can't be determined. Ventricular rate is 20 to 40 beats/minute.
P wave: Absent.

PR interval: Unmeasurable because of the absent P wave.
QRS complex: Because of abnormal ventricular depolarization, the QRS complex has a duration longer than 0.12 second, with a wide and bizarre configuration.
T wave: The T wave is abnormal. Deflection usually occurs in the opposite direction from that of the QRS complex.
QT interval: Usually prolonged.
Other: Idioventricular rhythm commonly occurs with third-degree atrioventricular block.

SIGNS AND SYMPTOMS

The patient with continuous idioventricular rhythm is generally symptomatic because of the marked reduction in cardiac output that occurs with the arrhythmia. Blood pressure may be difficult or impossible to auscultate or pal-

Transcutaneous pacemaker

Transcutaneous pacing, also referred to as *external pacing* or *noninvasive pacing*, involves the delivery of electrical impulses through externally applied cutaneous electrodes. The electrical impulses are conducted through an intact chest wall using skin electrodes placed either in anterior-posterior or sternal-apex positions. (An anterior-posterior placement is shown here.)

Transcutaneous pacing is the initial pacing method of choice in emergency situations because it's the least invasive technique and it can be instituted quickly.

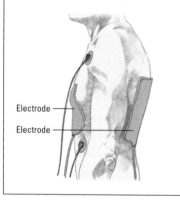

Electrode

Electrode

pate. The patient may experience dizziness, light-headedness, syncope, or loss of consciousness.

INTERVENTIONS
Treatment should be initiated immediately to increase the patient's heart rate, improve cardiac output, and establish a normal rhythm. Atropine may be administered to increase the heart rate.

If atropine isn't effective or if the patient develops hypotension or other signs of clinical instability, a pacemaker may be needed to reestablish a heart rate that provides enough cardiac output to perfuse organs properly. A transcutaneous pacemaker may be used in an emergency until a temporary or transvenous pacemaker can be inserted. (See *Transcutaneous pacemaker.*)

Remember that the goal of treatment doesn't include suppressing the idioventricular rhythm because it acts as a safety mechanism to protect the heart from ventricular standstill. Idioventricular rhythm should never be treated with lidocaine or other antiarrhythmics that would suppress the escape beats.

Patients with idioventricular rhythm need continuous ECG monitoring and constant assessment until treatment restores hemodynamic stability. Keep atropine and pacemaker equipment available at the bedside. Enforce bed rest until an effective heart rate has been maintained and the patient is clinically stable.

Be sure to tell the patient and family members about the serious nature of this arrhythmia and the treatment it requires. If the patient needs a permanent pacemaker, teach the patient and family how it works, how to recognize problems, when to contact the physician, and how pacemaker function will be monitored.

Ventricular tachycardia

VT, also called *V-tach,* occurs when three or more PVCs strike in a row and the ventricular rate exceeds 100 beats/ minute. This life-threatening arrhyth-

Recognizing ventricular tachycardia

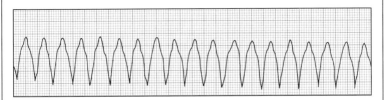

This rhythm strip illustrates ventricular tachycardia.

- *Rhythm:* regular
- *Rate:* 187 beats/minute
- *P wave:* absent
- *PR interval:* unmeasurable
- *QRS complex:* 0.24 second; wide and bizarre

- *T wave:* opposite direction of QRS complex
- *QT interval:* unmeasurable
- *Other:* none

mia usually precedes ventricular fibrillation and sudden cardiac death, especially in patients who aren't in a health care facility.

VT is an extremely unstable rhythm and may be sustained or non-sustained. When it occurs in short, paroxysmal bursts lasting under 30 seconds and causing few or no symptoms, it's called *non-sustained.* When the rhythm is sustained, however, it requires immediate treatment to prevent death, even in patients initially able to maintain adequate cardiac output. (See *Recognizing ventricular tachycardia.*)

CAUSES

This arrhythmia usually results from increased myocardial irritability, which may be triggered by enhanced automaticity, reentry within the Purkinje system, or by PVCs occurring during the downstroke of the preceding T wave.

Causes of VT include:
- myocardial ischemia
- MI
- coronary artery disease
- valvular heart disease
- heart failure
- cardiomyopathy
- electrolyte imbalances such as hypokalemia
- drug intoxication from procainamide, quinidine, or cocaine.

CLINICAL SIGNIFICANCE

VT is significant because of its unpredictability and potential for causing death. A patient may be hemodynamically stable, with a normal pulse and blood pressure; clinically unstable, with hypotension and poor peripheral pulses; or unconscious, without respirations or pulse.

Because of the reduced ventricular filling time and the drop in cardiac out-

WARNING

Recognizing torsades de pointes

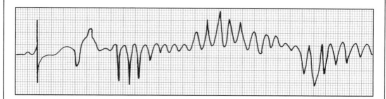

Characteristics of torsades de pointes:

- *Rhythm:* atrial rhythm — can't be determined; ventricular rhythm — regular or irregular
- *Rate:* atrial rate — can't be determined; ventricular rate — 150 to 250 beats/minute
- *P wave:* not identifiable because it's buried in the QRS complex
- *PR interval:* not applicable because P wave can't be identified

- *QRS complex:* usually wide with a phasic variation in its electrical polarity, shown by complexes that point downward for several beats, and vice versa
- *T wave:* not discernible
- *QT interval:* prolonged
- *Other:* may be paroxysmal, starting and stopping suddenly

---

put that occurs with this arrhythmia, the patient's condition can quickly deteriorate to ventricular fibrillation and complete cardiovascular collapse.

ECG CHARACTERISTICS

Rhythm: Atrial rhythm can't be determined. Ventricular rhythm is usually regular but may be slightly irregular.
Rate: Atrial rate can't be determined. Ventricular rate is usually rapid (100 to 250 beats/minute).
P wave: The P wave is usually absent. It may be obscured by the QRS complex; P waves are dissociated from the QRS complexes. Retrograde and upright P waves may be present.
PR interval: Unmeasurable because the P wave can't be seen in most cases.

QRS complex: Duration is greater than 0.12 second; it usually has a bizarre appearance, with increased amplitude. QRS complexes in monomorphic VT have a uniform shape. In polymorphic VT, the shape of the QRS complex constantly changes.
T wave: If the T wave is visible, it occurs opposite the QRS complex.
QT interval: Unmeasurable.
Other: Ventricular flutter and torsades de pointes are two variations of this arrhythmia. Torsades de pointes is a special variation of polymorphic VT. (See *Recognizing torsades de pointes*.) Although a relatively rare occurrence, torsades de pointes is sometimes difficult to distinguish from ventricular flutter. (See *Distinguishing ventricular flutter from torsades de pointes*.)

LOOK-ALIKES

Distinguishing ventricular flutter from torsades de pointes

Torsades de pointes is a variant form of ventricular tachycardia, with a rapid ventricular rate that varies between 250 and 350 beats/minute. It's characterized by QRS complexes that gradually change back and forth, with the amplitude of each successive complex gradually increasing and decreasing. This results in an overall outline of the rhythm commonly described as *spindle shaped.*

Ventricular flutter, although rarely recognized, results from the rapid, regular, repetitive beating of the ventricles. It's produced by a single ventricular focus firing at a rapid rate of 250 to 350 beats/minute. The hallmark of this arrhythmia is its smooth sine-wave appearance.

The illustrations shown here highlight key differences in the two arrhythmias.

Ventricular flutter
• smooth, sine-wave appearance

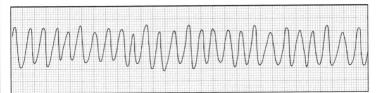

Torsades de pointes
• spindle-shaped appearance

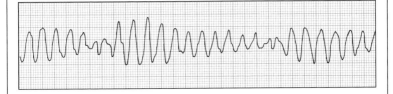

Distinguishing ventricular tachycardia from supraventricular tachycardia

Differentiating ventricular tachycardia (VT) from supraventricular tachycardia (SVT) with aberrancy is difficult. Careful assessment of a 12-lead ECG or rhythm strip can help you differentiate the arrhythmia with 90% accuracy.

Begin by looking at the deflection—negative or positive. Then use the following illustrations to guide your assessment. If the QRS complex is wide and mostly negative in deflection in V_1 or MCL_1, use these clues.

Ventricular tachycardia

- If the QRS complex has an R wave ≥ 0.04 second, a slurred S (shown below, shaded), or a notched S (shown below at right) on the downstroke, suspect VT.

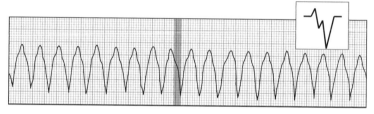

Supraventricular tachycardia

- If the QRS complex has an R wave ≤ 0.04 second and a swift, straight S on the downstroke (shown below, shaded, and below right), suspect SVT with aberrancy.

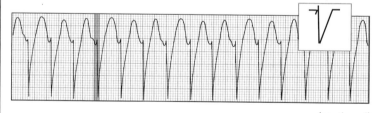

(continued)

Sometimes distinguishing VT from supraventricular tachycardia can be extremely challenging, especially in the setting of aberrant ventricular conduction. (See *Distinguishing ventricular tachycardia from supraventricular tachycardia.*)

SIGNS AND SYMPTOMS

Although some patients have only minor symptoms initially, they still require rapid intervention to prevent cardiovascular collapse. Most patients with VT have weak or absent pulses. Low cardiac output will cause hypotension and a decreased level of con-

Distinguishing ventricular tachycardia from supraventricular tachycardia (continued)

If the QRS complex is wide and mostly positive in deflection in V_1 or MCL_1, use these clues.

Ventricular tachycardia
• If the QRS complex is biphasic, suspect VT.

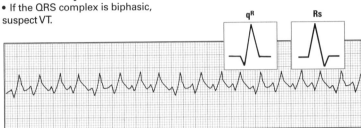

Supraventricular tachycardia
• If the beat is triphasic, similar to a right bundle-branch block, suspect SVT with aberrancy.

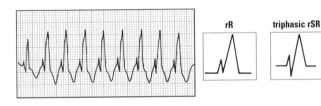

Other clues you can use if the QRS complex is wide and mostly positive in deflection in lead V_1 or MCL_1 include the following:

If the QRS complex is tall and shaped like rabbit ears, with the left peak taller than the right, suspect VT.

If the QRS complex is monophasic, suspect VT.

(continued)

Distinguishing ventricular tachycardia from supraventricular tachycardia *(continued)*

If you still have trouble differentiating the rhythm, look at V_6 or MCL_6.

If the S wave is larger than the R wave, suspect VT.

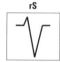

If any Q wave is present, suspect VT.

Other general criteria can also help you differentiate VT from SVT with aberrancy.
• A QRS complex > 0.14 second suggests VT.
• A regular, wide, complex rhythm suggests VT.

• An irregular, wide, complex rhythm suggests SVT with aberrancy.
• Concordant V leads (the QRS complex either mainly positive or mainly negative in all V leads) suggest VT.
• Atrioventricular dissociation suggests VT.

sciousness, quickly leading to unresponsiveness if left untreated. VT may prompt angina, heart failure, or a substantial decrease in organ perfusion.

INTERVENTIONS

Treatment depends on the patient's clinical status. Is the patient conscious? Does the patient have spontaneous respirations? Is a palpable carotid pulse present?

Patients with pulseless VT are treated the same as those with ventricular fibrillation and require immediate defibrillation. Treatment for patients with a detectable pulse depends on whether they're stable or unstable.

Unstable patients generally have ventricular rates greater than 150 beats/minute and have serious signs and symptoms related to the tachycardia, which may include hypotension, shortness of breath, chest pain, or altered consciousness. These patients are usually treated with immediate synchronized cardioversion.

A clinically stable patient with wide-complex VT and no signs of heart failure is treated differently. Treatment for these patients is determined by whether the VT is monomorphic or polymorphic, whether the patient has normal or impaired cardiac function, and whether the baseline QT interval is normal or prolonged. (See *Stable monomorphic or polymorphic ventricular tachycardia algorithm.*)

Patients with chronic, recurrent episodes of VT unresponsive to drug therapy may need an implanted cardioverter-defibrillator (ICD). This device is a permanent solution to recurrent episodes of VT. (See *Understanding the implantable cardioverter-defibrillator,* page 114.)

A 12-lead ECG and all other available clinical information is critical for establishing a specific diagnosis in a stable patient with wide QRS complex

Stable monomorphic or polymorphic ventricular tachycardia algorithm

Cardioversion is an appropriate, immediate treatment for any stable ventricular tachycardia (VT). Alternatives to this treatment depend on the type of VT, the patient's cardiac function, and the configuration of the QT interval. In monomorphic VT, QRS complexes keep the same form or appearance. In polymorphic VT, QRS complexes occur in more than one form, varying in appearance.

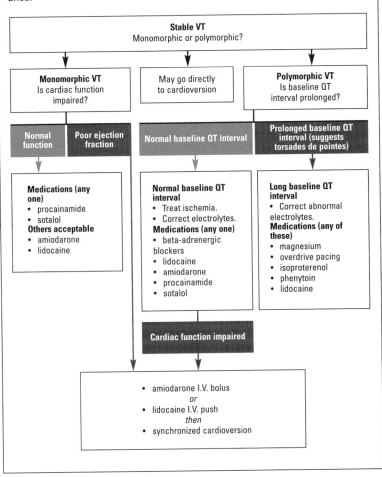

Understanding the implantable cardioverter-defibrillator

The implantable cardioverter-defibrillator (ICD) has a programmable pulse generator and lead system that monitors the heart's activity, detects ventricular arrhythmias and other tachyarrhythmias, and responds with appropriate therapies. The range of therapies includes antitachycardia and antibradycardia pacing, cardioversion, and defibrillation. Newer defibrillators can also pace the atrium and the ventricle.

Implantation of the ICD is similar to that of a permanent pacemaker. The cardiologist positions the lead (or leads) transvenously in the endocardium of the right ventricle (and the right atrium, if both chambers require pacing). The lead connects to a generator box implanted in the right or left upper chest near the clavicle.

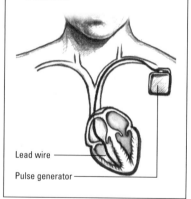

Lead wire

Pulse generator

tachycardia of unknown type. If a definitive diagnosis of supraventricular tachycardia or VT can't be established,

the patient's treatment should be guided by whether cardiac function is preserved (ejection fraction greater than 40%).

Be sure to teach patients and families about the serious nature of this arrhythmia and the need for prompt treatment. If your stable patient is undergoing electrical cardioversion, inform him that he'll be given a sedative, and possibly an analgesic, prior to the procedure.

If a patient will be discharged with an ICD or a prescription for long-term antiarrhythmics, ensure that family members know how to use the emergency medical system and how to perform CPR.

Ventricular fibrillation

Ventricular fibrillation, commonly called *V-fib* or *VF*, is characterized by a chaotic, disorganized pattern of electrical activity. The pattern arises from electrical impulses coming from multiple ectopic pacemakers in the ventricles.

The arrhythmia produces no effective ventricular mechanical activity or contractions and no cardiac output. Untreated VF is the most common cause of sudden cardiac death in people outside of a health care facility. (See *Recognizing ventricular fibrillation*.)

CAUSES
Causes of VF include:
- coronary artery disease
- myocardial ischemia
- MI

Recognizing ventricular fibrillation

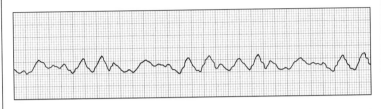

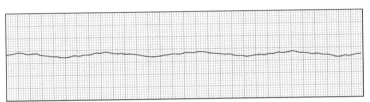

Characteristics of ventricular fibrillation (VF):

- *Rhythm:* chaotic
- *Rate:* can't be determined
- *P wave:* absent
- *PR interval:* unmeasurable
- *QRS complex:* indiscernible
- *T wave:* indiscernible
- *QT interval:* not applicable

- *Other:* the presence of large fibrillatory waves indicates coarse VF (as shown in the first ECG strip); the presence of small fibrillatory waves indicates fine VF (as shown in the second ECG strip)

- untreated VT
- underlying heart disease
- acid-base imbalance
- electric shock
- severe hypothermia
- drug toxicity, including digoxin, quinidine, and procainamide
- electrolyte imbalances, such as hypokalemia, hyperkalemia, and hypercalcemia.

CLINICAL SIGNIFICANCE

With VF, the ventricular muscle quivers, replacing effective muscular contraction with completely ineffective

contraction. Cardiac output falls to zero and, if allowed to continue, leads to ventricular standstill and death.

ECG CHARACTERISTICS

Rhythm: Atrial rhythm can't be determined. Ventricular rhythm has no pattern or regularity. Ventricular electrical activity appears as fibrillatory waves with no recognizable pattern.

Rate: Atrial and ventricular rates can't be determined.

P wave: Can't be determined.

PR interval: Can't be determined.

QRS complex: Duration can't be determined.

T wave: Can't be determined.

QT interval: Not applicable.

Other: Coarse fibrillatory waves are generally associated with greater chances of successful electrical cardioversion than smaller amplitude waves. Fibrillatory waves become finer as hypoxemia and acidosis progress, making the VF more resistant to defibrillation.

SIGNS AND SYMPTOMS

The patient in VF is in full cardiac arrest, unresponsive, and without a detectable blood pressure or central pulses. Whenever you see an ECG pattern resembling VF, check the patient immediately and initiate definitive treatment.

INTERVENTIONS

When faced with a rhythm that appears to be VF, always assess the patient first. Other events can mimic VF on an ECG strip, including interference from an electric razor, shivering, or seizure activity.

Immediate defibrillation is the most effective treatment for VF. CPR must be performed until the defibrillator arrives to preserve oxygen supply to the brain and other vital organs. Drugs such as epinephrine and vasopressin may be used for persistent VF if an initial three attempts at electrical defibrillation fail to correct the arrhythmia. Antiarrhythmic agents, such as amiodarone and magnesium, may also be considered. (See *Ventricular fibrillation and pulseless ventricular tachycardia algorithm.*)

In defibrillation, two electrode pads are applied to the chest wall. Current is then directed through the pads and, subsequently, the patient's chest and heart. The current causes the myocardium to completely depolarize, which, in turn, encourages the SA node to resume normal control of the heart's electrical activity.

One electrode pad is placed to the right of the upper sternum, and one is placed over the fifth or sixth intercostal space at the left anterior axillary line. During cardiac surgery, internal paddles are placed directly on the myocardium.

Automated external defibrillators (AEDs) are increasingly being used, especially in the out-of-hospital setting, to provide early defibrillation. After a patient is confirmed to be unresponsive, breathless, and pulseless, the AED power is turned on and the electrode pads and cables attached. The AED can analyze the patient's cardiac rhythm and provide the caregiver with step-by-step instructions on how to proceed. These defibrillators can be used by people without medical experience as long as they're trained in the proper use of the device. (See *Automated external defibrillator,* page 118.)

For the patient in VF, successful resuscitation requires rapid recognition of the problem and prompt defibrillation. Many health care facilities and emergency medical systems have established protocols so that health care workers can initiate prompt treatment. Make sure you know the location of your facility's emergency equipment, and make sure you know how to use it.

You'll also need to teach the patient and family how to use the emergency medical system following discharge from the facility. Family members may need instruction in CPR. Teach them

Ventricular fibrillation and pulseless ventricular tachycardia algorithm

Ventricular fibrillation (VF) and pulseless ventricular tachycardia (VT) require aggressive, systematic treatment. Follow the algorithm below for patients with these arrhythmias.

Primary ABCD survey
Focus: basic cardiopulmonary resuscitation and defibrillation

- Check responsiveness.
- Activate emergency response system.
- Call for defibrillator.
- **A** Airway: Open the airway.
- **B** Breathing: Provide positive-pressure ventilations.

- **C** Circulation: Give chest compressions.
- **D** Defibrillation: Assess for VF or pulseless VT and defibrillate up to three times (200 joules, 200 to 300 joules, 360 joules, or equivalent biphasic), if necessary.

Rhythm after first three cardioversions?

Persistent or recurrent VF or VT

Secondary ABCD survey
Focus: more advanced assessments and treatments

- **A** Airway: Insert airway device as soon as possible.
- **B** Breathing: Confirm airway device placement by exam plus confirmation device.
- **B** Breathing: Secure airway device: purpose-made tube holders preferred.
- **B** Breathing: Confirm effective oxygenation and ventilation.

- **C** Circulation: Establish I.V. access.
- **C** Circulation: Identify rhythm and monitor.
- **C** Circulation: Administer drugs appropriate for rhythm and condition.
- **D** Differential Diagnosis: Search for and treat identified reversible causes.

- epinephrine I.V. push; repeat every 3 to 5 minutes
  or
- vasopressin I.V.; single dose, one time only

Resume attempts to defibrillate.
1 × 360 joules (or equivalent biphasic) within 30 to 60 seconds

Consider antiarrhythmics.

- amiodarone (class IIb intervention)
- lidocaine (indeterminate)
- magnesium (IIb if hypomagnesemic state)

- procainamide (IIb for intermittent or recurrent VF or VT)
- Consider buffers.

Resume attempts to defibrillate.

Automated external defibrillator

Automated external defibrillators (AEDs) vary with the manufacturer, but the basic components of each device are similar. This illustration shows a typical AED and how to place electrodes properly.

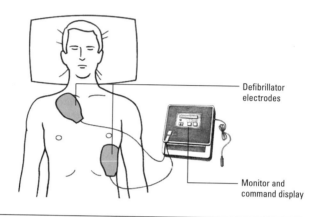

Defibrillator electrodes

Monitor and command display

about long-term therapies that help prevent recurrent episodes of VF, including antiarrhythmic drug therapy and ICDs.

Asystole

Ventricular asystole, also called *asystole* and *ventricular standstill,* is the absence of discernable electrical activity in the ventricles. Although some electrical activity may be evident in the atria, these impulses aren't conducted to the ventricles. (See *Recognizing asystole.*)

Asystole usually results from a prolonged period of cardiac arrest without effective resuscitation. It's important to distinguish asystole from fine VF, which is managed differently. There-

fore, asystole must be confirmed in more than one ECG lead.

CAUSES
Possible reversible causes of asystole include:
- hypovolemia
- MI (coronary thrombosis)
- severe electrolyte disturbances, especially hyperkalemia and hypokalemia
- massive pulmonary embolism
- hypoxia
- severe, uncorrected acid-base disturbances, especially metabolic acidosis
- drug overdose
- hypothermia
- cardiac tamponade
- tension pneumothorax.

CLINICAL SIGNIFICANCE
Without ventricular electrical activity, ventricular contractions can't occur. As

WARNING

 Recognizing asystole

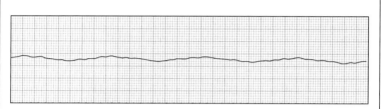

Characteristics of asystole:

- *Rhythm:* atrial rhythm — usually indiscernible; no ventricular rhythm
- *Rate:* atrial rate — usually indiscernible; no ventricular rate
- *P wave:* may be present
- *PR interval:* unmeasurable

- *QRS complex:* absent, or occasional escape beats
- *T wave:* absent
- *QT interval:* unmeasurable
- *Other:* absence of electrical activity in the ventricles results in a nearly flat line

a result, cardiac output drops to zero and vital organs are no longer perfused. Asystole has been called the *arrhythmia of death* and is typically considered to be a confirmation of death, rather than an arrhythmia to be treated.

The patient with asystole is completely unresponsive, without spontaneous respirations or pulse (cardiopulmonary arrest). Without immediate initiation of CPR and rapid identification and treatment of the underlying cause, the condition quickly becomes irreversible.

ECG CHARACTERISTICS

Rhythm: Atrial rhythm is usually indiscernible; no ventricular rhythm is present.
Rate: Atrial rate is usually indiscernible; no ventricular rate is present.
P wave: May be present.
PR interval: Unmeasurable.

QRS complex: Absent or occasional escape beats.
T wave: Absent.
QT interval: Unmeasurable.
Other: On a rhythm strip, asystole looks like a nearly flat line (except for changes caused by chest compressions during CPR). In a patient with a pacemaker, pacer spikes may be evident on the strip but no P wave or QRS complex occurs in response to the stimulus.

SIGNS AND SYMPTOMS

The patient will be unresponsive and have no spontaneous respirations, discernible pulse, or blood pressure.

INTERVENTIONS

Immediate treatment for asystole includes effective CPR, supplemental oxygen, and advanced airway control with tracheal intubation. Resuscitation should be attempted unless evidence

Asystole algorithm

Few patients with asystole survive. The treatment goal is to reestablish a heart rhythm. Treatment includes pacing and appropriate medications to stimulate impulse conduction. Use the following algorithm to guide treatment of the patient with asystole.

Primary ABCD survey
Focus: basic cardiopulmonary resuscitation and defibrillation

- Check responsiveness.
- Activate emergency response system.
- Call for defibrillator.
- **A** Airway: Open the airway.
- **B** Breathing: Provide positive-pressure ventilations.
- **C** Circulation: Give chest compressions.

- **C** Circulation: Confirm true asystole.
- **D** Defibrillation: Assess for ventricular fibrillation (VF) or pulseless ventricular tachycardia (VT); defibrillate, if indicated.
- Rapid scene survey: Any evidence personnel should not attempt resuscitation?

Secondary ABCD survey
Focus: more advanced assessments and treatments

- **A** Airway: Place airway device as soon as possible.
- **B** Breathing: Confirm airway device placement by exam plus confirmation device.
- **B** Breathing: Secure airway device: purpose-made tube holders preferred.
- **B** Breathing: Confirm effective oxygenation and ventilation.

- **C** Circulation: Confirm true asystole.
- **C** Circulation: Establish I.V. access.
- **C** Circulation: Identify rhythm on monitor.
- **C** Circulation: Give medications appropriate for rhythm and condition.
- **D** Differential Diagnosis: Search for and treat identified reversible causes.

Transcutaneous pacing
If considered, perform immediately.

---

epinephrine I.V. push; repeat every 3 to 5 minutes

---

atropine I.V. push

Asystole persists
Withhold or cease resuscitation efforts?

- Consider quality of resuscitation?
- Atypical clinical features present?
- Support for cease-efforts protocols in place?

Pulseless electrical activity

Pulseless electrical activity (PEA) defines a group of arrhythmias characterized by the presence of some type of electrical activity but no detectable pulse. Although organized electrical depolarization occurs, no synchronous shortening of the myocardial fibers occurs. As a result, no mechanical activity or contractions take place. Included in the PEA category are electromechanical dissociation (EMD), pseudo-EMD, idioventricular rhythms, and ventricular escape rhythms.

Causes

The most common causes of PEA include hypovolemia, hypoxia, acidosis, tension pneumothorax, cardiac tamponade, massive pulmonary embolism, hypothermia, hyperkalemia and hypokalemia, massive acute myocardial infarction, and overdoses of drugs such as tricyclic antidepressants.

Treatment

Rapid identification and treatment of underlying reversible causes is critical for treating PEA. For example, hypovolemia is treated with volume expansion. Tension pneumothorax is treated with needle decompression.

Institute cardiopulmonary resuscitation, tracheal intubation, and I.V. administration of epinephrine. Atropine may be given if the PEA rate is slow.

---

exists that these efforts shouldn't be initiated, such as when a do-not-resuscitate order is in effect. (See *Asystole algorithm*.)

Remember to verify the presence of asystole by checking more than one ECG lead. Priority must also be given to searching for and treating identified potentially reversible causes. Early transcutaneous pacing may be considered, and I.V. epinephrine and atropine is administered as ordered.

Be aware that pulseless electrical activity can also lead to asystole. Know how to recognize this problem and treat it. (See *Pulseless electrical activity*.)

With persistent asystole despite appropriate management, consideration should be given to terminating resuscitation.

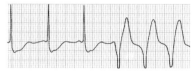

SkillCheck

1. Using the 8-step method for ECG analysis, interpret the following arrhythmia.

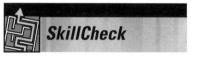

Answer:
Rhythm: Atrial and ventricular rhythms are irregular.
Rate: Atrial rate is 40 beats/minute; ventricular rate is 70 beats/minute.
P wave: Normal configuration, except absent with four aberrant beats.
PR interval: 0.14 second with normal beats; absent with aberrant beats.
QRS complex: 0.08 second with nor-

mal beats; 0.14 second with aberrant beats.

T wave: Normal configuration; deflection opposite QRS complex with aberrant beats.

QT interval: 0.48 second with normal beats; 0.40 second with aberrant beats.

Other: None.

Interpretation: Sinus rhythm with three-beat run of VT.

2. Using the 8-step method for ECG analysis, interpret the following arrhythmia.

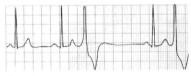

Answer:

Rhythm: Atrial and ventricular rhythms are irregular.

Rate: Atrial rate is 40 beats/minute; ventricular rate is 60 beats/minute.

P wave: Normal size and configuration.

PR interval: 0.16 second.

QRS complex: 0.06 second with normal complexes; 0.22 second with wide complexes.

T wave: Normal configuration, except with aberrant beats T wave deflected in opposite direction of QRS complex.

QT interval: 0.36 second with normal complexes; 0.44 second with wide complexes.

Other: None.

Interpretation: Normal sinus rhythm with uniform ventricular bigeminy.

3. Using the 8-step method for ECG analysis, interpret the following arrhythmia.

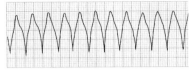

Answer:

Rhythm: Atrial rhythm can't be determined; ventricular rhythm is regular.

Rate: Atrial rate can't be determined; ventricular rate is 160 beats/minute.

P wave: Absent.

PR interval: Unmeasurable.

QRS complex: 0.18 second; wide and bizarre.

T wave: Opposite direction of QRS complex.

QT interval: Unmeasurable.

Other: None.

Interpretation: VT.

4. Using the 8-step method for ECG analysis, interpret the following arrhythmia.

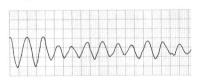

Answer:

Rhythm: Atrial rhythm can't be determined; ventricular rhythm is rapid, chaotic, and irregular.

Rate: Atrial and ventricular rates can't be determined.

P wave: Indiscernible.

PR interval: Indiscernible.

QRS complex: Indiscernible.

T wave: Indiscernible.

QT interval: Indiscernible.

Other: None.

Interpretation: Coarse ventricular fibrillation.

5. Using the 8-step method for ECG analysis, interpret the following arrhythmia.

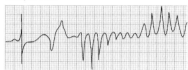

Answer:

Rhythm: Atrial rhythm can't be determined; ventricular rhythm is irregular.

Rate: Atrial rate can't be determined; ventricular rate is 250 beats/minute.

P wave: Normal configuration in first beat; can't be identified in aberrant beats.

PR interval: 0.14 second on first beat, then can't be determined.

QRS complex: Wide; complexes deflect downward, then upward, then downward again; duration varies.

T wave: Distorted.

QT interval: 0.72 second with first beat; then can't be determined.

Other: None.

Interpretation: Torsades de pointes.

7 Atrioventricular blocks

Atrioventricular (AV) heart block refers to an interruption or delay in the conduction of electrical impulses between the atria and the ventricles. The block can occur at the AV node, the bundle of His, or the bundle branches. When the site of block is the bundle of His or the bundle branches, the block is referred to as *infranodal AV block*. AV block can be partial (first or second degree) or complete (third degree).

The heart's electrical impulses normally originate in the sinoatrial (SA) node, so when those impulses are blocked at the AV node, atrial rates are often normal (60 to 100 beats/minute). The clinical significance of the block depends on the number of impulses completely blocked and the resulting ventricular rate. A slow ventricular rate can decrease cardiac output and cause symptoms such as light-headedness, hypotension, and confusion.

CAUSES OF AV BLOCK

A variety of factors may lead to AV block, including underlying heart conditions, use of certain drugs, congenital anomalies, and conditions that disrupt the cardiac conduction system.

Typical causes of AV block include:
■ myocardial ischemia, which impairs cellular function so that cells repolarize more slowly or incompletely. The injured cells, in turn, may conduct impulses slowly or inconsistently. Relief of the ischemia may restore normal function to the AV node.
■ myocardial infarction (MI), in which cellular necrosis or death occurs. If the necrotic cells are part of the conduction system, they may no longer conduct impulses and a permanent AV block occurs.
■ excessive serum levels of, or an exaggerated response to, a drug. This response can cause AV block or increase the likelihood that a block will develop. The drugs may increase the refractory period of a portion of the conduction system. Although many antiarrhythmics can have this effect, the drugs more commonly known to cause or exacerbate AV blocks include digoxin, beta-adrenergic blockers, and calcium channel blockers.
■ lesions, including calcium and fibrotic lesions, along the conduction pathway.
■ congenital anomalies such as congenital ventricular septal defects that involve cardiac structures and affect the conduction system. Anomalies of the conduction system, such as an AV node that doesn't conduct impulses, can also occur in the absence of structural defects.

AV block can also be caused by inadvertent damage to the heart's conduction system during cardiac surgery. Damage is most likely to occur in operations involving the mitral or tricuspid valve or in the closure of a ventricular septal defect. If the injury involves tissues adjacent to the surgical site and the conduction system isn't physically disrupted, the block may be only temporary. If a portion of the conduction system itself is severed, permanent block results.

Similar disruption of the conduction system can occur from a procedure called *radiofrequency ablation.* In this invasive procedure, a transvenous catheter is used to locate the area in the heart that participates in initiating or perpetuating certain tachyarrhythmias. Radiofrequency energy is then delivered to the myocardium through this catheter to produce a small area of necrosis at that spot. The damaged tissue can no longer cause or participate in the tachyarrhythmia. If the energy is delivered close to the AV node, bundle of His, or bundle branches, however, AV block can result.

CLASSIFICATION OF AV BLOCK

AV blocks are classified according to the site of block and the severity of the conduction abnormality. The sites of AV block include the AV node, bundle of His, and bundle branches.

Severity of AV block is classified in degrees: first-degree AV block; second-degree AV block, type I (Wenckebach or Mobitz I); second-degree AV block, type II (Mobitz II) AV block; and third-degree (complete) AV block. The classification system for AV blocks aids in the determination of the patient's treatment and prognosis.

First-degree atrioventricular block

First-degree AV block occurs when there's a delay in the conduction of electrical impulses from the atria to the ventricles. This delay usually occurs at the level of the AV node, but it may also be infranodal. First-degree AV block is characterized by a PR interval greater than 0.20 second. This interval usually remains constant beat to beat. Electrical impulses are conducted through the normal conduction pathway. However, conduction of these impulses takes longer than normal.

CAUSES

First-degree AV block may result from myocardial ischemia or MI, myocarditis, or degenerative changes in the heart associated with aging. The condition may also be caused by drugs, such as digoxin, calcium channel blockers, and beta-adrenergic blockers.

CLINICAL SIGNIFICANCE

First-degree AV block may cause no symptoms in a healthy person. The arrhythmia may be transient, especially if it occurs secondary to drugs or ischemia early in the course of an MI. The presence of first-degree block, the least dangerous type of AV block, indicates a delay in the conduction of electrical impulses through the normal conduction pathway. In general, a rhythm strip with this block looks like normal sinus rhythm except that the PR interval is longer than normal.

Recognizing first-degree atrioventricular block

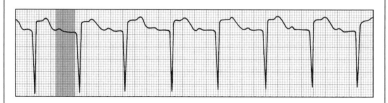

This rhythm strip illustrates first-degree atrioventricular block.

- *Rhythm:* regular
- *Rate:* 75 beats/minute
- *P wave:* normal
- *PR interval:* 0.32 second; greater than 0.20 second (see shaded area)
- *QRS complex:* 0.08 second
- *T wave:* normal
- *QT interval:* 0.40 second
- *Other:* PR interval — prolonged but constant

Because first-degree AV block can progress to a more severe type of AV block, the patient's cardiac rhythm should be monitored for changes. (See *Recognizing first-degree atrioventricular block.*)

ECG CHARACTERISTICS

Rhythm: Atrial and ventricular rhythms are regular.

Rate: Atrial and ventricular rates are the same and within normal limits.

P wave: Normal size and configuration; each P wave followed by a QRS complex.

PR interval: Prolonged (greater than 0.20 second) but constant.

QRS complex: Duration usually remains within normal limits if the conduction delay occurs in the AV node. If the QRS duration exceeds 0.12 second, the conduction delay may be in the His-Purkinje system.

T wave: Normal size and configuration unless the QRS complex is prolonged.

QT interval: Usually within normal limits.

Other: None.

SIGNS AND SYMPTOMS

The patient's pulse rate will usually be normal and the rhythm will be regular. Most patients with first-degree AV block are asymptomatic because cardiac output isn't significantly affected. If the PR interval is extremely long, a longer interval between S_1 and S_2 may be noted on cardiac auscultation.

INTERVENTIONS

Treatment generally focuses on identification and correction of the underlying cause. For example, if a drug is causing the AV block, the dosage may be reduced or the drug discontinued. Close monitoring can help detect progression of first-degree AV block to a more serious form of block.

Evaluate a patient with first-degree AV block for underlying causes that can be corrected, such as drugs or myocardial ischemia. Observe the electrocardiogram (ECG) for progression of the block to a more severe form. Administer digoxin, calcium channel blockers, and beta-adrenergic blockers cautiously.

Second-degree atrioventricular block

Second-degree AV block occurs when some of the electrical impulses from the AV node are blocked and some are conducted through normal conduction pathways. Second-degree AV block is subdivided into type I second-degree AV block and type II second-degree AV block.

TYPE I SECOND-DEGREE AV BLOCK

Also called *Wenckebach* or *Mobitz I block,* type I second-degree AV block occurs when each successive impulse from the SA node is delayed slightly longer than the previous impulse. (See *Recognizing type I second-degree atrioventricular block,* page 128.) This pattern of progressive prolongation of the PR interval continues until an impulse fails to be conducted to the ventricles.

Usually only a single impulse is blocked from reaching the ventricles, and following this nonconducted P wave or dropped beat, the pattern is repeated. This repetitive sequence of

two or more consecutive beats followed by a dropped beat results in "group beating." Type I second-degree AV block generally occurs at the level of the AV node.

Causes

Type I second-degree AV block frequently results from increased parasympathetic tone or the effects of certain drugs. Coronary artery disease, inferior-wall MI, and rheumatic fever may increase parasympathetic tone and result in the arrhythmia. It may also be due to cardiac medications, such as beta-adrenergic blockers, digoxin, and calcium channel blockers.

Clinical significance

Type I second-degree AV block may occur normally in an otherwise healthy person. Almost always transient, this type of block usually resolves when the underlying condition is corrected. Although an asymptomatic patient with this block has a good prognosis, the block may progress to a more serious form, especially if it occurs early in an MI.

ECG characteristics

Rhythm: Atrial rhythm is regular, and the ventricular rhythm is irregular. The R-R interval shortens progressively until a P wave appears without a QRS complex. The cycle is then repeated.
Rate: The atrial rate exceeds the ventricular rate because of the nonconducted beats, but both usually remain within normal limits.
P wave: Normal size and configuration; each P wave is followed by a QRS complex except for the blocked P wave.

Recognizing type I second-degree atrioventricular block

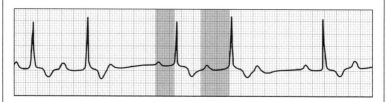

This rhythm strip illustrates type I second-degree atrioventricular block.

- *Rhythm:* atrial—regular; ventricular—irregular
- *Rate:* atrial—80 beats/minute; ventricular—50 beats/minute
- *P wave:* normal
- *PR interval:* progressively prolonged (see shaded areas)
- *QRS complex:* 0.08 second
- *T wave:* normal
- *QT interval:* 0.46 second
- *Other:* Wenckebach pattern of grouped beats; the PR interval gets progressively longer until a QRS complex is dropped

PR interval: The PR interval is progressively longer with each cycle until a P wave appears without a QRS complex. The variation in delay from cycle to cycle is typically slight. The PR interval after the nonconducted beat is shorter than the interval preceding it. The phrase commonly used to describe this pattern is *long, longer, dropped.*

QRS complex: Duration usually remains within normal limits because the block commonly occurs at the level of the AV node. The complex is periodically absent.

T wave: Normal size and configuration, but its deflection may be opposite that of the QRS complex.

QT interval: Usually within normal limits.

Other: The arrhythmia is usually distinguished by group beating, referred to as the *footprints of Wenckebach.*

K. Frederik Wenckebach was a Dutch internist who, at the turn of the century and long before the introduction of the ECG, described the two forms of what's now known as *second-degree AV block* by analyzing waves in the jugular venous pulse. Following the introduction of the ECG, German cardiologist Woldemar Mobitz clarified Wenckebach's findings, identifying two types of second-degree AV block, type I and type II.

Signs and symptoms

Usually asymptomatic, a patient with type I second-degree AV block may show signs and symptoms of decreased cardiac output, such as light-headedness or hypotension. Symptoms may be especially pronounced if the ventricular rate is slow.

Interventions

Treatment is rarely needed because the patient is generally asymptomatic. For a patient with serious signs and symptoms related to a low heart rate, atropine may be used to improve AV node conduction. A transcutaneous pacemaker may be required for a symptomatic patient until the arrhythmia resolves. (See *Bradycardia algorithm,* page 46.)

When caring for a patient with this block, assess the tolerance for the rhythm and the need for treatment to improve cardiac output. Evaluate the patient for possible causes of the block, including the use of certain medications or the presence of myocardial ischemia.

Check the ECG frequently to see if a more severe type of AV block develops. Make sure the patient has a patent I.V. line. Provide patient teaching about a temporary pacemaker if indicated.

TYPE II SECOND-DEGREE AV BLOCK

Type II second-degree AV block (also known as *Mobitz II block*) is less common than type I, but more serious. It occurs when impulses from the SA node occasionally fail to conduct to the ventricles. This form of second-degree AV block occurs below the level of the AV node, either at the bundle of His, or more commonly at the bundle branches.

One of the hallmarks of this type of block is that, unlike type I second-degree AV block, the PR interval doesn't lengthen before a dropped beat. (See *Recognizing type II second-degree atrioventricular block,* page 130.) In addition, more than one nonconducted beat can occur in succession.

Causes

Unlike type I second-degree AV block, type II second-degree AV block rarely results from increased parasympathetic tone or drug effect. Because the arrhythmia is usually associated with organic heart disease, it's usually associated with a poorer prognosis, and complete heart block may develop.

Type II second-degree AV block is commonly caused by an anterior-wall MI, degenerative changes in the conduction system, or severe coronary artery disease. The arrhythmia indicates a conduction disturbance at the level of the bundle of His or bundle branches.

Clinical significance

Unlike type I second-degree AV block, type II second-degree AV block rarely results from increased parasympathetic tone or drug effect. As a result, this type of block is usually associated with a poorer prognosis and a greater probability that complete heart block may develop.

In type II second-degree AV block, the ventricular rate tends to be slower than in type I. In addition, cardiac output tends to be lower and symptoms are more likely to appear, particularly if the sinus rhythm is slow and the ratio of conducted beats to dropped beats is low such as 2:1.

ECG characteristics

Rhythm: The atrial rhythm is regular. The ventricular rhythm can be regular or irregular. Pauses correspond to the dropped beat. When the block is intermittent or when the conduction ratio is variable, the rhythm is often irregular. When a constant conduction ratio oc-

Recognizing type II second-degree atrioventricular block

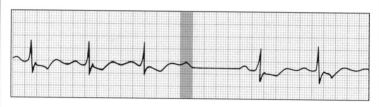

This rhythm illustrates type II second-degree atrioventricular block.

- *Rhythm:* atrial—regular; ventricular—irregular
- *Rate:* atrial—60 beats/minute; ventricular—50 beats/minute
- *P wave:* normal
- *PR interval:* 0.28 second; the PR interval is constant for the conducted beats

- *QRS complex:* 0.10 second
- *T wave:* normal
- *QT interval:* 0.60 second
- *Other:* PR and R-R intervals don't vary before a dropped beat (see shaded area), so no warning occurs

curs, for example, 2:1 or 3:1, the rhythm is regular.

Rate: The atrial rate is usually within normal limits. The ventricular rate, slower than the atrial rate, may be within normal limits.

P wave: The P wave is normal in size and configuration, but some P waves aren't followed by a QRS complex. The R-R interval containing a nonconducted P wave equals two normal R-R intervals.

PR interval: The PR interval is within normal limits or prolonged but generally always constant for the conducted beats. It may be shortened if following a nonconducted beat.

QRS complex: Duration is within normal limits if the block occurs at the bundle of His. If the block occurs at the bundle branches, however, the QRS will be widened and display the features of bundle-branch block. The complex is absent periodically.

T wave: Usually of normal size and configuration.

QT interval: Usually within normal limits.

Other: The PR and R-R intervals don't vary before a dropped beat, so no warning occurs. For a dropped beat to occur, there must be complete block in one bundle branch with intermittent interruption in conduction in the other bundle as well. As a result, this type of second-degree AV block is commonly associated with a wide QRS complex. However, when the block occurs at the bundle of His, the QRS may be narrow

Distinguishing nonconducted premature atrial contractions from type II second-degree atrioventricular block

An isolated P wave that doesn't conduct through to the ventricle (P wave without a QRS complex following it; see shaded areas) may occur with a nonconducted premature atrial contraction (PAC) or may indicate type II second-degree atrioventricular (AV) block. Mistakenly identifying AV block as nonconducted PACs may have serious consequences. The latter is generally benign; the former can be life-threatening.

Nonconducted PAC

If the P-P interval, including the extra P wave, isn't constant, it's a nonconducted PAC.

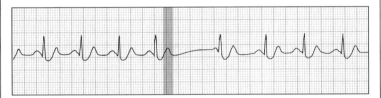

Type II second-degree AV block

If the P-P interval is constant, including the extra P wave, it's type II second-degree AV block.

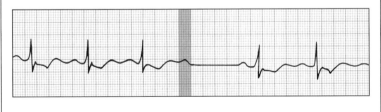

since ventricular conduction is undisturbed in beats that aren't blocked.

It may be difficult to distinguish nonconducted premature atrial contractions from type II second-degree AV block. (See *Distinguishing nonconducted premature atrial contractions from type II second-degree atrioventricular block*.)

Signs and symptoms

Most patients who experience occasional dropped beats remain asymptomatic as long as cardiac output is maintained. As the number of dropped beats increases, the patient may experience signs and symptoms of decreased cardiac output, including fatigue, dyspnea, chest pain, or light-headedness. On physical examination, you may note hypotension and a slow pulse, with a regular or irregular rhythm.

Interventions

If the patient doesn't experience serious signs and symptoms related to the low heart rate, the patient may be prepared for transvenous pacemaker insertion. Alternatively, the patient may be continuously monitored, with a transcutaneous pacemaker readily available.

If the patient is experiencing serious signs and symptoms due to bradycardia, treatment goals include improving cardiac output by increasing the heart rate. Intravenous atropine, transcutaneous pacing, I.V. dopamine, or I.V. epinephrine may be used to increase cardiac output. (See *Bradycardia algorithm,* page 46.)

Because this form of second-degree AV block occurs below the level of the AV node — either at the bundle of His or, more commonly, at the bundle branches — transcutaneous pacing should be initiated quickly, when indicated. For this reason, type II second-degree AV block also may require placement of a permanent pacemaker. A temporary pacemaker may be used until a permanent pacemaker can be inserted.

When caring for a patient with type II second-degree block, assess tolerance for the rhythm and the need for treatment to improve cardiac output. Evaluate for possible correctable causes such as ischemia.

Keep the patient on bed rest, if indicated, to reduce myocardial oxygen demands. Administer oxygen therapy as ordered. Observe the patient's cardiac rhythm for progression to a more severe form of AV block. Teach the patient and family about the use of pacemakers if the patient requires one.

Third-degree atrioventricular block

Also called *complete heart block* or *AV dissociation,* third-degree AV block indicates the complete absence of impulse conduction between the atria and ventricles. In complete heart block, the atrial rate is generally equal to or faster than the ventricular rate.

Third-degree AV block may occur at the level of the AV node, the bundle of His, or the bundle branches. The patient's treatment and prognosis vary depending on the anatomic level of the block.

When third-degree AV block occurs at the level of the AV node, ventricular depolarization is typically initiated by a junctional escape pacemaker. This pacemaker is usually stable with a rate of 40 to 60 beats/minute. (See *Recognizing third-degree atrioventricular block.*) The sequence of ventricular depolarization is usually normal because the block is located above the bifurcation of the bundle of His, which results in a normal-appearing QRS complex.

On the other hand, when third-degree AV block occurs at the infranodal level, a block involving the right and left bundle branches is most com-

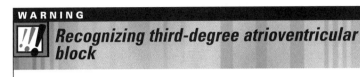

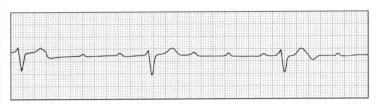

This rhythm strip illustrates third-degree atrioventricular block:

- *Rhythm:* regular
- *Rate:* atrial— 90 beats/minute; ventricular—30 beats/minute
- *P wave:* normal
- *PR interval:* varied
- *QRS complex:* 0.16 second
- *T wave:* normal
- *QT interval:* 0.56 second
- *Other:* P waves occur without a QRS complex

monly the cause. In this case, extensive disease exists in the infranodal conduction system, and the only available escape mechanism is located distal to the site of block in the ventricle. This unstable, ventricular escape pacemaker has a slow intrinsic rate of under 40 beats/minute. Because these depolarizations originate in the ventricle, the QRS complex will have a wide and bizarre appearance.

CAUSES

Third-degree AV block occurring at the anatomic level of the AV node can result from increased parasympathetic tone associated with inferior wall MI, AV node damage, or toxic effects of drugs, such as digoxin and propranolol.

Third-degree AV block occurring at the infranodal level is frequently associated with extensive anterior MI. It

generally isn't the result of increases in parasympathetic tone or drug effect.

CLINICAL SIGNIFICANCE

Third-degree AV block occurring at the AV node, with a junctional escape rhythm, is usually transient and generally associated with a favorable prognosis. In third-degree AV block at the infranodal level, however, the pacemaker is unstable and episodes of ventricular asystole are common. Third-degree AV block at this level is generally associated with a less favorable prognosis.

Because the ventricular rate in third-degree AV block can be slow and the decrease in cardiac output so significant, the arrhythmia usually results in a life-threatening situation. In addition, the loss of AV synchrony results in the loss of atrial kick, which further decreases cardiac output.

ECG CHARACTERISTICS

Rhythm: Atrial and ventricular rhythms are usually regular.

Rate: Acting independently, the atria, generally under the control of the SA node, tend to maintain a regular rate of 60 to 100 beats/minute. The atrial rate exceeds the ventricular rate. With intranodal block, the ventricular rate is usually 40 to 60 beats/minute (a junctional escape rhythm). With infranodal block, the ventricular rate is usually below 40 beats/minute (a ventricular escape rhythm).

P wave: The P wave is normal in size and configuration. Some P waves may be buried in QRS complexes or T waves.

PR interval: Not applicable or measurable because the atria and ventricles are depolarized from different pacemakers and beat independently of each other (AV dissociation).

QRS complex: Configuration depends on the location of the escape mechanism and origin of ventricular depolarization. When the block occurs at the level of the AV node or bundle of His, the QRS complex will appear normal. When the block occurs at the level of the bundle branches, the QRS will be widened.

T wave: Normal size and configuration unless the QRS complex originates in the ventricle.

QT interval: May be within normal limits.

Other: None.

SIGNS AND SYMPTOMS

Most patients with third-degree AV block experience significant signs and symptoms, including severe fatigue, dyspnea, chest pain, light-headedness, changes in mental status, and changes in the level of consciousness. Hypotension, pallor, and diaphoresis may also occur. The peripheral pulse rate will be slow, but the rhythm will be regular.

A few patients will be relatively free of symptoms, complaining only that they can't tolerate exercise and that they're typically tired for no apparent reason. The severity of symptoms depends to a large extent on the resulting ventricular rate and the patient's ability to compensate for decreased cardiac output.

INTERVENTIONS

If the patient is experiencing serious signs and symptoms related to the low heart rate, or if the patient's condition seems to be deteriorating, interventions may include transcutaneous pacing or I.V. atropine, dopamine, or epinephrine.

Asymptomatic patients in third-degree AV block should be prepared for insertion of a transvenous temporary pacemaker until a decision is made about the need for a permanent pacemaker. If symptoms develop, a transcutaneous pacemaker should be used until the transvenous pacemaker is placed.

Because third-degree AV block occurring at the infranodal level is usually associated with extensive anterior MI, patients are more likely to have permanent third-degree AV block, which most likely requires insertion of a permanent pacemaker.

Third-degree AV block occurring at the anatomic level of the AV node can result from increased parasympathetic tone associated with an inferior wall MI. As a result, the block is more likely to be short-lived. In these patients, the decision to insert a permanent pacemaker is often delayed to assess how well the conduction system recovers.

When caring for a patient with third-degree heart block, immediately assess the patient's tolerance of the rhythm and the need for interventions to support cardiac output and relieve symptoms. Make sure that the patient has a patent I.V. line. Administer oxygen therapy as ordered. Evaluate for possible correctable causes of the arrhythmia, such as drugs or myocardial ischemia. Minimize the patient's activity and maintain bed rest.

SkillCheck

1. Using the 8-step method for ECG analysis, interpret the following arrhythmia.

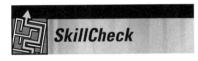

Answer:
Rhythm: Atrial and ventricular rhythms are regular with the exception of the ectopic beat.
Rate: Atrial rate is 50 beats/minute; ventricular rate is 60 beats/minute.
P wave: Normal size and configuration except absent with ectopic beat.
PR interval: 0.22 second with normal P waves.
QRS complex: 0.06 second with normal beat; 0.20 second with aberrant beat.
T wave: Normal configuration, except with aberrant beat's T wave deflected in opposite direction of QRS complex.

QT interval: 0.58 second.
Other: None.
Interpretation: First-degree AV block with one premature ventricular contraction.

2. Using the 8-step method for ECG analysis, interpret the following arrhythmia.

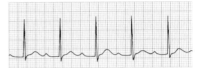

Answer:
Rhythm: Atrial and ventricular rhythms are regular.
Rate: Atrial and ventricular rates are 75 beats/minute.
P wave: Normal size and configuration.
PR interval: 0.34 second.
QRS complex: 0.08 second.
T wave: Normal configuration.
QT interval: 0.42 second.
Other: None.
Interpretation: Normal sinus rhythm with first-degree AV block.

3. Using the 8-step method for ECG analysis, interpret the following arrhythmia.

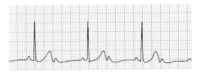

Answer:
Rhythm: Atrial and ventricular rhythms are regular.
Rate: Atrial rate is 100 beats/minute; ventricular rate is 50 beats/minute.
P wave: Normal size and configuration; two P waves for each QRS complex.
PR interval: 0.14 second.

QRS complex: 0.06 second.
T wave: Normal configuration.
QT interval: 0.44 second.
Other: None.
Interpretation: Type II (Mobitz II) second-degree AV block.

4. Using the 8-step method for ECG analysis, interpret the following arrhythmia.

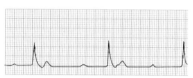

Answer:
Rhythm: Atrial and ventricular rhythms are regular.
Rate: Atrial rate is 75 beats/minute; ventricular rate is 41 beats/minute.
P wave: Normal size; no constant relationship to QRS complex.
PR interval: Not applicable.
QRS complex: 0.16 second; wide and bizarre.
T wave: Second beat distorted by P wave; other beats with normal configuration.
QT interval: 0.42 second.
Other: None.
Interpretation: Third-degree AV block (complete heart block).

5. Using the 8-step method for ECG analysis, interpret the following arrhythmia.

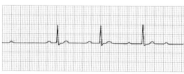

Answer:
Rhythm: Atrial and ventricular rhythms are irregular.
Rate: Atrial rate is 70 beats/minute;

ventricular rate is 50 beats/minute.
P wave: Normal size and configuration.
PR interval: Progressively lengthens with each cycle, until a QRS complex is dropped.
QRS complex: 0.06 second.
T wave: Normal configuration.
QT interval: 0.32 second.
Other: None.
Interpretation: Type I (Mobitz I or Wenckebach) second-degree AV block.

Disorder, drug, and surgical effects

This chapter reviews electrocardiogram (ECG) characteristics associated with selected disorders and drugs. ECG characteristics of patients who have undergone certain surgical procedures will also be addressed, including the insertion of a pacemaker, an implantable cardioverter-defibrillator (ICD), and a ventricular assist device (VAD) as well as cardiac transplantation.

Rhythm strips of patients with electrolyte imbalances, such as hyperkalemia, hypokalemia, hypercalcemia, and hypocalcemia, frequently show distinctive patterns. Patients taking drugs, such as digoxin, may also exhibit characteristic appearances on an ECG that can provide early warnings of drug toxicity. By recognizing some of these variations early, you may be able to identify and treat potentially dangerous conditions before they become serious.

Keep in mind, however, that the patient's ECG is only part of the clinical picture. Additional information, such as the patient's medical history, findings on physical examination, and additional diagnostic studies, will be necessary to confirm an initial diagnosis based on ECG analysis.

Electrolyte imbalances

Potassium and calcium ions play a major role in the electrical activity of the heart. Depolarization results from the exchange of these ions across the cell membrane. Changes in ion concentration can affect the heart's electrical activity and, as a result, the patient's ECG. This section examines ECG effects from high and low potassium and calcium levels.

Hyperkalemia

Potassium, the most plentiful intracellular cation (positively charged electrolyte), contributes to many important cellular functions. Most of the body's potassium content is located in the cells. The intracellular fluid (ICF) concentration of potassium is 150 to 160 mEq/L; the extracellular fluid (ECF) concentration, 3.5 to 4.5 mEq/L. Many symptoms associated with potassium imbalance result from changes in this ratio of ICF to ECF potassium concentration. Hyperkalemia is generally defined as an elevation of serum potassium above 5.5 mEq/L.

ECG effects of hyperkalemia

The classic and most striking ECG feature of hyperkalemia is tall, peaked T waves. This rhythm strip shows a typical peaked T wave (shaded area).

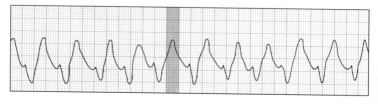

CAUSES

■ An increased intake of potassium, including excessive dietary intake and I.V. administration of penicillin G, potassium supplements, or banked whole blood.

■ A shift of potassium from ICF to ECF occurring with changes in cell membrane permeability or damage, including extensive surgery, burns, massive crush injuries, cell hypoxia, acidosis, and insulin deficiency.

■ Decreased renal excretion, including renal failure, decreased production and secretion of aldosterone, Addison's disease, and use of potassium-sparing diuretics.

CLINICAL SIGNIFICANCE

When extracellular potassium concentrations increase without a significant change in intracellular potassium concentrations, the cell becomes less negative, or partially depolarized, and the resting cell membrane potential decreases. Mild elevations in extracellular potassium result in cells that repolarize faster and are more irritable.

More critical elevations in extracellular potassium result in an inability of cells to repolarize and respond to elec-

trical stimuli. Cardiac standstill, or asystole, is the most serious consequence of severe hyperkalemia.

ECG CHARACTERISTICS

Rhythm: Atrial and ventricular rhythms are regular.

Rate: Atrial and ventricular rates are within normal limits.

P wave: In mild hyperkalemia, the amplitude is low; in moderate hyperkalemia, P waves are wide and flattened; in severe hyperkalemia, the P wave may be indiscernible.

PR interval: Normal or prolonged; unmeasurable if P wave can't be detected.

QRS complex: Widened because ventricular depolarization takes longer.

ST segment: May be elevated in severe hyperkalemia.

T wave: Tall, peaked; the classic and most striking feature of hyperkalemia.

QT interval: Shortened.

Other: Intraventricular conduction disturbances commonly occur. (See *ECG effects of hyperkalemia.*)

SIGNS AND SYMPTOMS

Mild hyperkalemia may cause neuro-muscular irritability, including restlessness, intestinal cramping, diarrhea, and tingling lips and fingers. Severe hyperkalemia may cause loss of muscle tone, muscle weakness, and paralysis.

INTERVENTIONS

Treatment depends upon the severity of hyperkalemia and the patient's signs and symptoms. The underlying cause must be identified and the extracellular potassium concentration brought back to normal. Drug therapy to normalize potassium levels includes calcium gluconate to decrease neuromuscular irritability, insulin and glucose to facilitate the entry of potassium into the cell, and sodium bicarbonate to correct metabolic acidosis.

Oral or rectal administration of cation exchange resins, such as sodium polystyrene sulfonate, may be used to exchange sodium for potassium in the intestine. In the setting of renal failure or severe hyperkalemia, dialysis may be necessary to remove excess potassium. The patient's serum potassium levels should be monitored closely until they return to normal, and arrhythmias should be identified and managed appropriately.

Hypokalemia

Hypokalemia, or potassium deficiency, occurs when the ECF concentration of potassium drops below 3.5 mEq/L, usually indicating a loss of total body potassium. The concentration of ECF potassium is so small that even minor changes in ECF potassium affect resting membrane potential.

CAUSES

Factors contributing to the development of hypokalemia include increased loss of body potassium, increased entry of potassium into cells, and reduced potassium intake. Shifts in potassium from the extracellular space to the intracellular space may be caused by alkalosis, especially respiratory alkalosis. Intracellular uptake of potassium is also increased by catecholamines. Although rare, dietary deficiency in the elderly may contribute to hypokalemia. The condition is also seen in patients with alcoholism or anorexia nervosa.

GI and renal disorders are the most common causes of potassium loss from body stores. GI losses of potassium are associated with laxative abuse, intestinal fistulae or drainage tubes, diarrhea, vomiting, and continuous nasogastric drainage.

Renal loss of potassium is related to increased secretion of potassium by the distal tubule. Diuretics, a low serum magnesium concentration, and excessive aldosterone secretion may cause urinary loss of potassium. In addition, several antibiotics, including gentamicin and amphotericin B, are known to cause hypokalemia.

CLINICAL SIGNIFICANCE

When extracellular potassium levels decrease rapidly and intracellular potassium concentration doesn't change, the resting membrane potential becomes more negative and the cell membrane becomes hyperpolarized. The cardiac effects of hypokalemia are related to these changes in membrane excitability. Ventricular repolarization

ECG effects of hypokalemia

As the serum potassium concentration drops, the T wave becomes flat and a U wave appears (shaded area). The rhythm strip below shows typical ECG effects of hypokalemia.

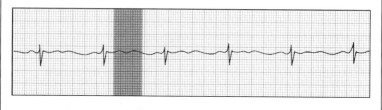

is delayed because potassium contributes to the repolarization phase of the action potential. Hypokalemia can cause dangerous ventricular arrhythmias and increases the risk of digoxin toxicity.

ECG CHARACTERISTICS
Rhythm: Atrial and ventricular rhythms are regular.
Rate: Atrial and ventricular rates are within normal limits.
P wave: Usually normal size and configuration but may become peaked in severe hypokalemia.
PR interval: May be prolonged.
QRS complex: Within normal limits or possibly widened; prolonged in severe hypokalemia.
QT interval: Usually indiscernible as the T wave flattens.
ST segment: Depressed.
T wave: Amplitude is decreased. The T wave becomes flat as the potassium level drops. In severe hypokalemia, it flattens completely and may become inverted. The T wave may also fuse with an increasingly prominent U wave.

Other: Amplitude of the U wave is increased, becoming more prominent as hypokalemia worsens and fusing with the T wave. (See *ECG effects of hypokalemia*.)

SIGNS AND SYMPTOMS
The most common symptoms of hypokalemia are caused by neuromuscular and cardiac effects, including smooth muscle atony, skeletal muscle weakness, and cardiac arrhythmias. Loss of smooth muscle tone results in constipation, intestinal distention, nausea, vomiting, anorexia, and paralytic ileus. Skeletal muscle weakness occurs first in the larger muscles of the arms and legs and eventually affects the diaphragm, causing respiratory arrest.

Cardiac effects of hypokalemia include arrhythmias, such as bradycardia, atrioventricular (AV) block, and paroxysmal atrial tachycardia (PAT). Delayed depolarization results in characteristic changes on the ECG.

INTERVENTIONS
The underlying causes of hypokalemia should be identified and corrected. Acid-base imbalances should be cor-

rected, potassium losses replaced, and further losses prevented. Encourage intake of foods and fluids rich in potassium. Oral or I.V. potassium supplements may be administered. The patient's serum potassium levels should be monitored closely until they return to normal, and cardiac arrhythmias should be identified and managed appropriately.

Hypercalcemia

Most of the body's calcium stores (99%) are located in bone. The remainder is found in the plasma and body cells. Approximately 50% of plasma calcium is bound to plasma proteins. About 40% is found in the ionized or free form.

Calcium plays an important role in myocardial contractility. Ionized calcium is more important than plasma-bound calcium in physiologic functions. Hypercalcemia is usually defined as a serum calcium concentration greater than 12 mg/dl.

CAUSES

The most common causes of hypercalcemia include excess vitamin D intake; bone metastasis and calcium resorption associated with cancers of the breast, prostate, and cervix; hyperparathyroidism; sarcoidosis; and many parathyroid hormone (PTH)-producing tumors.

CLINICAL SIGNIFICANCE

In hypercalcemia, calcium is found inside cells in greater abundance than normal. The cell membrane becomes refractory to depolarization as a result of a more positive action potential.

This loss of cell membrane excitability causes many of the cardiac symptoms seen in patients with hypercalcemia.

Both ventricular depolarization and repolarization are accelerated. The patient may experience bradyarrhythmias and varying degrees of AV block.

ECG CHARACTERISTICS

Rhythm: Atrial and ventricular rhythms are regular.
Rate: Atrial and ventricular rates are within normal limits, but bradycardia can occur.
P wave: Normal size and configuration.
PR interval: May be prolonged.
QRS complex: Within normal limits, but may be prolonged.
QT interval: Shortened.
ST segment: Shortened.
T wave: Normal size and configuration; may be depressed.
Other: None. (See *ECG effects of hypercalcemia,* page 142.)

SIGNS AND SYMPTOMS

Common signs and symptoms of hypercalcemia include anorexia, nausea, constipation, lethargy, fatigue, and weakness. Behavioral changes may also occur. Renal calculi may form as precipitates of calcium salts, and impaired renal function frequently occurs. A reciprocal decrease in serum phosphate levels often accompanies elevated levels of serum calcium.

INTERVENTIONS

Treatment of hypercalcemia focuses on identifying and managing the underlying cause and is guided by the severity of the patient's symptoms. The administration of oral phosphate is usually effective as long as renal function is normal. In more critical situations, I.V. ad-

ECG effects of hypercalcemia

Increased serum concentrations of calcium cause shortening of the QT interval (shaded area). The rhythm strip shown here illustrates this key ECG finding in hypercalcemia.

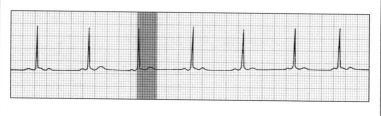

ministration of large volumes of normal saline solution may enhance renal excretion of calcium. On occasion, corticosteroids and mithramycin (a cytotoxic drug) have been used to treat hypercalcemia.

Hypocalcemia

Hypocalcemia occurs when the serum calcium level is below 8.5 mg/dl and ionized levels are below 4.0 mg/dl.

CAUSES

Hypocalcemia may be related to decreases in PTH and vitamin D, inadequate intestinal absorption, blood administration, or deposition of ionized calcium into soft tissue or bone.

Inadequate dietary intake of green, leafy vegetables or dairy products may result in a nutritional deficiency of calcium. Excessive dietary intake of phosphorus binds with calcium and prevents calcium absorption. The citrate solution used in storing whole blood binds with calcium, frequently resulting in hypocalcemia. Pancreatitis decreases

ionized calcium, and neoplastic bone metastases decrease serum calcium levels.

Decreased intestinal absorption of calcium is caused by vitamin D deficiency, either from inadequate vitamin D intake or insufficient exposure to sunlight. Other causes of hypocalcemia include malabsorption of fats, removal of the parathyroid glands, metabolic or respiratory alkalosis, and hypoalbuminemia.

CLINICAL SIGNIFICANCE

Hypocalcemia causes an increase in neuromuscular excitability. Partial depolarization of nerves and muscle cells result from a decrease in threshold potential. As a result, a smaller stimulus is needed to initiate an action potential. Characteristic ECG changes are a result of prolonged ventricular depolarization and decreased cardiac contractility.

ECG CHARACTERISTICS

Rhythm: Atrial and ventricular rhythms are regular.
Rate: Atrial and ventricular rates are within normal limits.

ECG effects of hypocalcemia

Decreased serum concentrations of calcium prolong the QT interval, as shown (shaded area) in this rhythm strip.

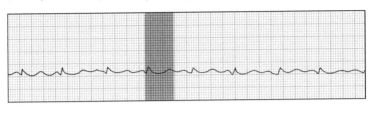

P wave: Normal size and configuration.
PR interval: Within normal limits.
QRS complex: Within normal limits.
QT interval: Prolonged.
ST segment: Prolonged.
T wave: Normal size and configuration, but may become flat or inverted.
Other: None. (See *ECG effects of hypocalcemia.*)

SIGNS AND SYMPTOMS

Symptoms of hypocalcemia include hyperreflexia, carpopedal spasm, confusion, and circumoral and digital paresthesias. Hyperactive bowel sounds and intestinal cramping may also occur. Severe symptoms include tetany, convulsions, respiratory arrest, and death. Clinical signs indicating hypocalcemia include Trousseau's sign and Chvostek's sign.

INTERVENTIONS

Treatment should focus on identifying and managing the underlying causes of hypocalcemia. Severe symptoms require emergency treatment with I.V. calcium gluconate. Serum calcium levels should be monitored and oral calcium replacement initiated when possi-

ble. Cardiac arrhythmias need to be identified and managed appropriately. Long-term management of hypocalcemia includes decreasing phosphate intake.

Cardiac drugs

Almost half a million Americans die each year from cardiac arrhythmias; countless others experience symptoms and lifestyle modifications. Along with other treatments, cardiac drugs can help alleviate symptoms, control heart rate and rhythm, decrease preload and afterload, and prolong life.

Antiarrhythmics affect the movement of ions across the cell membrane and alter the electrophysiology of the cardiac cell. These drugs are classified according to their effect on the cell's electrical activity (action potential) and their mechanism of action. Because the drugs can cause changes in the myocardial action potential, characteristic ECG changes can occur.

The classification system divides antiarrhythmic drugs into four major classes based on their dominant mecha-

ECG effects of class IA antiarrhythmics

Class IA antiarrhythmic drugs—including such drugs as quinidine and procainamide—affect the cardiac cycle in specific ways and lead to specific ECG
changes, as shown below. Class IA antiarrhythmics:
• block sodium influx during phase 0, which depresses the rate of depolarization
• prolong repolarization and the duration of the action potential
• lengthen the refractory period
• decrease contractility.

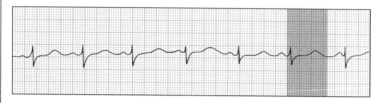

ECG characteristics (shaded area) of class IA antiarrhythmics:

• *QRS complex:* slightly widened   • *QT interval:* prolonged

---

nism of action: class I, class II, class
III, and class IV. Class I antiarrhythmics are further divided into class IA,
class IB, and class IC.

Certain antiarrhythmics can't be
classified specifically into one group.
For example, sotalol possesses characteristics of both class II and class III
drugs. Still, other drugs, such as adenosine, digoxin, atropine, epinephrine,
and magnesium, don't fit into the classification system at all. Despite its limi-
tations, the classification system is
helpful in understanding how antiarrhythmics prevent and treat arrhythmias.

This section reviews ECG changes
that result when patients take therapeutic doses of antiarrhythmics (separated
by classification) and digoxin. When
drug levels are toxic, ECG changes are
typically exaggerated.

Class I antiarrhythmics

Class I drugs block the influx of sodium into the cell during phase 0 of the
action potential. Because phase 0 is
also referred to as the sodium channel
or fast channel, these drugs may also
be called sodium channel blockers or
fast channel blockers. Class I drugs are
frequently subdivided into three
groups — A, B, and C — according to
their interactions with cardiac sodium
channels or the drug's effects on the
duration of the action potential.

CLASS IA

Class IA drugs include disopyramide,
procainamide, and quinidine. These
drugs lengthen the duration of the ac-

ECG effects of class IB antiarrhythmics

Class IB antiarrhythmic drugs — such as lidocaine and tocainide — may affect the QRS complex, as shown on the rhythm strip below. The drugs may also:
• block sodium influx during phase 0, which depresses the rate of depolarization
• shorten repolarization and the duration of the action potential
• suppress ventricular automaticity in ischemic tissue.

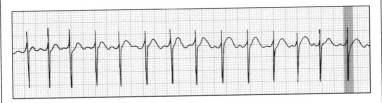

ECG characteristics of class IB antiarrhythmics:

• *PR interval:* may be prolonged

• *QRS complex:* slightly widened (shaded area)

tion potential, and their interaction with the sodium channels is classified as intermediate. As a result, conductivity is reduced and repolarization is prolonged.

ECG characteristics

Rhythm strip characteristics for a patient taking an antiarrhythmic vary according to the drug's classification. Variations for class IA drugs include:
■ *QRS complex:* Slightly widened; increased widening is an early sign of toxicity.
■ *T wave:* May be flattened or inverted.
■ *U wave:* May be present.
■ *QT interval:* Prolonged.

Because these drugs prolong the QT interval, the patient is prone to polymorphic ventricular tachycardia. (See *ECG effects of class IA antiarrhythmics.*)

CLASS IB

Class IB agents include phenytoin, lidocaine, and mexiletine. These agents interact rapidly with sodium channels, slowing phase 0 of the action potential and shortening phase 3. The drugs in this class are effective in suppressing ventricular ectopy.

ECG characteristics

When a patient is taking a class IB antiarrhythmic, check for these ECG changes:
■ *PR interval:* May be slightly shortened.
■ *QT interval:* Shortened. (See *ECG effects of class IB antiarrhythmics.*)

CLASS IC

Class IC agents, including flecainide and propafenone, may minimally increase or have no effect on the action potential duration. Class IC drugs inter-

ECG effects of class IC antiarrhythmics

Class IC antiarrhythmic drugs — including flecainide and propafenone — cause the effects shown below on an ECG by exerting particular actions on the cardiac cycle. Class IC antiarrhythmics block sodium influx during phase 0, which depresses the rate of depolarization. The drugs exert no effect on repolarization or the duration of the action potential.

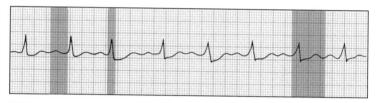

ECG characteristics of class IC antiarrhythmics:

- *PR interval:* prolonged (shaded area above left)
- *QRS complex:* widened (shaded area above center)
- *QT interval:* prolonged (shaded area above right)

---

act slowly with sodium channels. Phase 0 is markedly slowed and conduction is decreased.

These agents are generally reserved for refractory arrhythmias because they may cause or worsen arrhythmias.

ECG characteristics

When a patient is taking a class IC antiarrhythmic, look for the following ECG changes:

- *PR interval:* Prolonged.
- *QRS complex:* Widened.
- *QT interval:* Prolonged. (See *ECG effects of class IC antiarrhythmics.*)

Class II antiarrhythmics

Class II antiarrhythmics include drugs that reduce adrenergic activity in the heart. Beta-adrenergic antagonists, also called beta blockers, are class II antiarrhythmics and include such drugs as acebutolol and propranolol. Beta-adrenergic antagonists block beta receptors in the sympathetic nervous system. As a result, phase 4 depolarization is diminished, which leads to depressed automaticity of the sinoatrial (SA) node and increased atrial and AV node refractory periods.

Class II drugs are used to treat supraventricular and ventricular arrhythmias, especially those caused by excess circulating catecholamines.

ECG effects of class II antiarrhythmics

Class II antiarrhythmic drugs—including such beta-adrenergic blockers as propranolol, esmolol, and acebutolol—cause certain effects on an ECG (as shown here) by exerting particular actions on the cardiac cycle. Class II antiarrhythmics:
• depress sinoatrial node automaticity
• shorten the duration of the action potential
• increase the refractory period of atrial and atrioventricular junctional tissues, which slows conduction
• inhibit sympathetic activity.

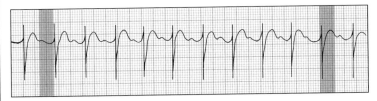

ECG characteristics of class II antiarrhythmics:

• *PR interval:* slightly prolonged (shaded area above left)

• *QT interval:* slightly shortened (shaded area above right)

Beta-adrenergic blockers are classified according to their effects. Beta$_1$-adrenergic blockers decrease heart rate, contractility, and conductivity. Beta$_2$-adrenergic blockers may cause vasoconstriction and bronchospasm because beta$_2$ receptors relax smooth muscle in the bronchi and blood vessels.

Beta-adrenergic blockers that block only beta$_1$ receptors are referred to as cardioselective. Those that have both beta$_1$- and beta$_2$-receptor activity are referred to as noncardioselective.

ECG CHARACTERISTICS

When a patient is taking a class II antiarrhythmic, you may see the following ECG changes:

■ *Rate:* Atrial and ventricular rates are decreased.

■ *PR interval:* Slightly prolonged.

■ *QT interval:* Slightly shortened. (See *ECG effects of class II antiarrhythmics.*)

Class III antiarrhythmics

Class III drugs prolong the action potential duration, which, in turn, prolongs the effective refractory period. Class III drugs are called potassium channel blockers because they block the movement of potassium during phase 3 of the action potential. Drugs in this class include amiodarone and ibutilide fumarate. All class III drugs have proarrhythmic potential.

ECG effects of class III antiarrhythmics

Class III antiarrhythmic drugs—including, amiodarone, sotalol, and ibutilide—affect the cardiac cycle and cause the effects shown here on an ECG. Class III antiarrhythmics:
• block potassium movement during phase 3
• increase the duration of the action potential
• prolong the effective refractory period.

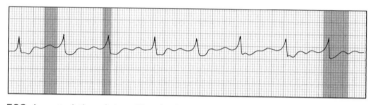

ECG characteristics of class III antiarrhythmics:

• *PR interval:* prolonged (shaded area above left)
• *QRS complex:* widened (shaded area above center)

• *QT interval:* prolonged (shaded area above right)

ECG CHARACTERISTICS

When a patient is taking a class III antiarrhythmic, you may see the following ECG changes:
▪ *PR interval:* Prolonged.
▪ *QRS complex:* Widened.
▪ *QT interval:* Prolonged. (See *ECG effects of class III antiarrhythmics.*)

Class IV antiarrhythmics

Class IV drugs block the movement of calcium during phase 2 of the action potential. Because phase 2 is also called the calcium channel or the slow channel, drugs that affect phase 2 are also known as calcium channel block-

ers or slow channel blockers. These drugs slow conduction and increase the refractory period of calcium-dependent tissues, including the AV node. Drugs in this class include verapamil and diltiazem.

ECG CHARACTERISTICS

When a patient is taking a class IV antiarrhythmic, check for these ECG changes:
▪ *Rate:* Atrial and ventricular rates are decreased.
▪ *PR interval:* Prolonged. (See *ECG effects of class IV antiarrhythmics.*)

ECG effects of class IV antiarrhythmics

Class IV antiarrhythmic drugs — including such calcium channel blockers as verapamil and diltiazem — affect the cardiac cycle in specific ways and may lead to a prolonged PR interval, as shown here. Class IV antiarrhythmics:
• block calcium movement during phase 2
• prolong the conduction time and increase the refractory period in the atrioventricular node
• decrease contractility.

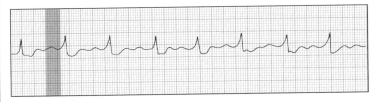

ECG characteristics of class IV antiarrhythmics:

• *PR interval:* prolonged (shaded area)

Digoxin

Digoxin, the most commonly used cardiac glycoside, works by inhibiting the enzyme adenosine triphosphatase. This enzyme is found in the plasma membrane and acts as a pump to exchange sodium ions for potassium ions. Inhibition of sodium-potassium–activated adenosine triphosphatase results in enhanced movement of calcium from the extracellular space to the intracellular space, thereby strengthening myocardial contractions.

The effects of digoxin on the electrical properties of the heart include direct and autonomic effects. Direct effects result in shortening of the action potential, which contributes to the shortening of atrial and ventricular refractoriness. Autonomic effects involve the sympathetic and parasympathetic systems. Vagal tone is enhanced, and conduction through the SA and AV nodes is slowed. The drug also exerts an antiarrhythmic effect.

Digoxin is indicated in the treatment of heart failure, paroxysmal supraventricular tachycardia, atrial fibrillation, and atrial flutter.

ECG CHARACTERISTICS

When a patient is taking digoxin, you may see the following ECG changes:
■ *Rate:* Atrial and ventricular rates are decreased.
■ *PR interval:* Shortened.
■ *T wave amplitude:* Decreased.
■ *ST segment:* Shortened and depressed. Sagging (scooping or sloping) of the segment is characteristic.
■ *QT interval:* Shortened due to the shortened ST segment.

ECG effects of digoxin

Digoxin affects the cardiac cycle in various ways and may lead to the ECG changes shown here.

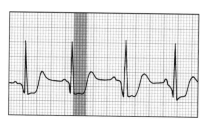

ECG characteristics of digoxin:

- *ST segment:* gradual sloping, causing ST-segment depression in the opposite direction of the QRS deflection (shaded area)
- *P wave:* may be notched

■ Digoxin has a very narrow window of therapeutic effectiveness and, at toxic levels, may cause numerous arrhythmias, including PAT with block, AV block, atrial and junctional tachyarrhythmias, and ventricular arrhythmias. (See *ECG effects of digoxin.*)

Surgeries

Certain surgical interventions produce distinctive ECG tracings. These interventions include various types of pacemakers, implantable cardioverter-defibrillators, ventricular assist devices, and transplanted hearts.

Pacemakers

A pacemaker is an artificial device that electrically stimulates the myocardium

to depolarize, initiating mechanical contractions. It works by generating an impulse from a power source and transmitting that impulse to the heart muscle. The impulse flows throughout the heart and causes the heart muscle to depolarize.

A pacemaker may be used when a patient has an arrhythmia, such as certain bradyarrhythmias and tachyarrhythmias, sick sinus syndrome, or an AV block. The device may be used as a temporary measure or a permanent one, depending on the patient's condition. Pacemakers are typically necessary following myocardial infarction or cardiac surgery.

This section examines how pacemakers work, ECG characteristics, types of pacemakers, synchronous and asynchronous pacing, biventricular pacemakers, description codes, pacing modes, assessment of pacemaker func-

Pacing leads

Pacing leads have either one electrode (unipolar) or two (bipolar). These illustrations show the difference between the two leads.

Unipolar lead
In a unipolar system, electrical current moves from the pulse generator through the leadwire to the negative pole. From there, it stimulates the heart and returns to the pulse generator's metal surface (the positive pole) to complete the circuit.

Bipolar lead
In a bipolar system, current flows from the pulse generator through the leadwire to the negative pole at the tip. At that point, it stimulates the heart and then flows back to the positive pole to complete the circuit.

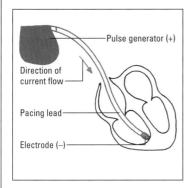

Pulse generator (+)
Direction of current flow
Pacing lead
Electrode (–)

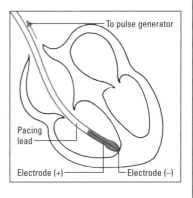

To pulse generator
Pacing lead
Electrode (+)
Electrode (–)

tion, troubleshooting a pacemaker, interventions, and patient teaching.

HOW PACEMAKERS WORK
A typical pacemaker has three main components: a pulse generator, battery, and microchip. The pulse generator contains the pacemaker's power source and circuitry. The lithium batteries in a permanent or implanted pacemaker serve as its power source and last about 10 years. A microchip in the device guides heart pacing.

A temporary pacemaker, which isn't implanted, is about the size of a small radio or telemetry box and is powered by alkaline batteries. These units also

contain a microchip and are programmed by a touch pad or dials.

An electrical stimulus from the pulse generator moves through wires, or pacing leads, to the electrode tips. The leads for a pacemaker, designed to stimulate a single heart chamber, are placed in either the atrium or the ventricle. For dual-chamber, or AV, pacing, the leads are placed in both chambers, usually on the right side of the heart. (See *Pacing leads*.)

The electrodes — one on a unipolar lead or two on a bipolar lead — send information about electrical impulses in the myocardium back to the pulse generator. The pulse generator senses

Pacemaker spikes

Pacemaker impulses—the stimuli that travel from the pacemaker to the heart—are visible on an electrocardiogram tracing as spikes. Large or small, pacemaker spikes appear above or below the isoelectric line. The rhythm strip below shows an atrial and a ventricular pacemaker spike.

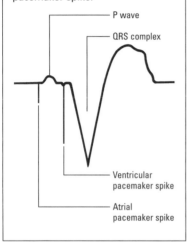

P wave

QRS complex

Ventricular pacemaker spike

Atrial pacemaker spike

the heart's electrical activity and responds according to how it was programmed.

A unipolar lead system is more sensitive to the heart's intrinsic electrical activity than a bipolar system. A bipolar system isn't as easily affected by electrical activity, such as skeletal muscle contraction or magnetic fields, originating outside the heart and the generator. A bipolar system is more difficult to implant, however.

ECG CHARACTERISTICS

The most prominent characteristic of a pacemaker on an ECG is the pacemak-

er spike. (See *Pacemaker spikes*.) It occurs when the pacemaker sends an electrical impulse to the heart muscle. The impulse appears as a vertical line, or spike. The collective group of spikes on an ECG is called pacemaker artifact.

Depending on the position of the electrode, the spike appears in different locations on the waveform:
- When the pacemaker stimulates the atria, the spike is followed by a P wave and the patient's baseline QRS complex and T wave. This series of waveforms represents successful pacing, or capture, of the myocardium. The P wave may appear different from the patient's normal P wave.
- When the ventricles are stimulated by a pacemaker, the spike is followed by a QRS complex and a T wave. The QRS complex appears wider than the patient's own QRS complex because of how the pacemaker depolarizes the ventricles.
- When the pacemaker stimulates both the atria and ventricles, the spike is followed by a P wave, then a spike, and then a QRS complex. Be aware that the type of pacemaker used and the patient's condition may affect whether every beat is paced.

PERMANENT PACEMAKERS

A permanent pacemaker is used to treat chronic heart conditions such as AV block. It's surgically implanted, usually under local anesthesia. The leads are placed transvenously, positioned in the appropriate chambers, and then anchored to the endocardium. (See *Placing a permanent pacemaker*.)

The generator is then implanted in a pocket made from subcutaneous tissue. The pocket is usually constructed under the clavicle. Most permanent pace-

Placing a permanent pacemaker

A surgeon who implants an endocardial pacemaker usually selects a transvenous route and begins lead placement by inserting a catheter percutaneously or by venous cutdown. Then, using fluoroscopic guidance, the catheter is threaded through the vein until the tip reaches the endocardium.

Atrial lead
For lead placement in the atrium, the tip must lodge in the right atrium or coronary sinus, as shown here. For placement in the ventricle, it must lodge within the right ventricular apex in one of the interior muscular ridges, or trabeculae.

Implanting the generator
When the lead is in the proper position, the pulse generator is secured in a subcutaneous pocket of tissue just below the clavicle. Changing the generator's battery or microchip circuitry requires only a shallow incision over the site and a quick component exchange.

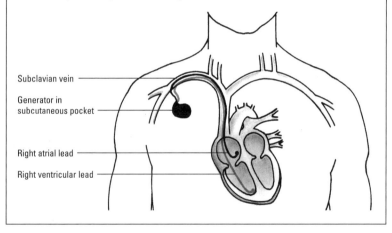

Subclavian vein

Generator in subcutaneous pocket

Right atrial lead

Right ventricular lead

makers are programmed before implantation. The programming sets the conditions under which the pacemaker functions and can be adjusted externally if necessary.

TEMPORARY PACEMAKERS
A temporary pacemaker is commonly inserted in an emergency. The patient may show signs of decreased cardiac output, such as hypotension or syncope. The temporary pacemaker supports the patient until the condition resolves.

A temporary pacemaker can also serve as a bridge until a permanent pacemaker is inserted. These pacemakers are used for patients with high-grade heart block, bradycardia, or low cardiac output. Several types of temporary pacemakers are available, including transvenous, epicardial, transcutaneous, and transthoracic.

Transvenous pacemakers

Physicians usually use the transvenous approach—inserting the pacemaker through a vein, such as the subclavian or internal jugular vein—when inserting a temporary pacemaker. The transvenous pacemaker is probably the most common and reliable type of temporary pacemaker. It's usually inserted at the bedside or in a fluoroscopy suite. The leadwires are advanced through a catheter into the right ventricle or atrium and then connected to the pulse generator.

Epicardial pacemakers

Epicardial pacemakers are commonly used for patients undergoing cardiac surgery. The tips of the leadwires are attached to the surface of the heart and then the wires are brought through the chest wall, below the incision. They're then attached to the pulse generator. The leadwires are usually removed several days after surgery or when the patient no longer requires them.

Transcutaneous pacemakers

Use of an external or transcutaneous pacemaker has become commonplace in the past several years. In this noninvasive method, one electrode is placed on the patient's anterior chest wall to the right of the upper sternum below the clavicle and a second electrode is applied to his back (anterior-posterior electrodes). One may also be placed to the left of the left nipple with the center of the electrode in the midaxillary line (also called the anterior-apex position). An external pulse generator then emits pacing impulses that travel through the skin to the heart muscle.

Transcutaneous pacing is a quick, effective method of pacing heart rhythm and is commonly used in emergencies until a transvenous pacemaker can be inserted. However, some patients may not be able to tolerate the irritating sensations produced from prolonged pacing at the levels needed to pace the heart externally. If hemodynamically stable, these patients may require sedation.

Transthoracic pacemakers

A transthoracic pacemaker is a type of temporary ventricular pacemaker only used during cardiac emergencies as a last resort. Transthoracic pacing requires insertion of a long needle into the right ventricle, using a subxyphoid approach. A pacing wire is then guided directly into the endocardium.

TEMPORARY PACEMAKER SETTINGS

A temporary pacemaker has several types of settings on the pulse generator. The rate control regulates how many impulses are generated in 1 minute and is measured in pulses per minute (ppm). The rate is usually set at 60 to 80 ppm. (See *Temporary pulse generator.*) The pacemaker fires if the patient's heart rate falls below the preset rate. The rate may be set higher if the patient has a tachyarrhythmia being treated with overdrive pacing.

The energy output of a pacemaker is measured in milliamperes (mA), a measurement that represents the stimulation threshold, or how much energy is required to stimulate the cardiac muscle to depolarize. The stimulation threshold is sometimes referred to as *energy required for capture.*

You can also program the pacemaker's sensitivity, measured in millivolts (mV). Most pacemakers allow the heart

Temporary pulse generator

The settings on a temporary pulse generator may be changed in a number of ways to meet the needs of a specific patient. The illustration below shows a single-chamber temporary pulse generator and brief descriptions of its various parts.

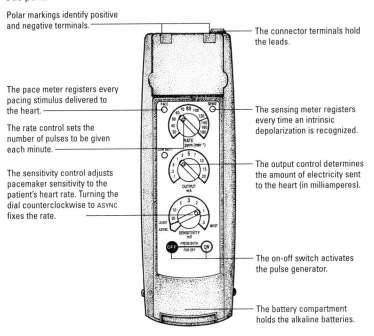

Polar markings identify positive and negative terminals.

The connector terminals hold the leads.

The pace meter registers every pacing stimulus delivered to the heart.

The rate control sets the number of pulses to be given each minute.

The sensing meter registers every time an intrinsic depolarization is recognized.

The sensitivity control adjusts pacemaker sensitivity to the patient's heart rate. Turning the dial counterclockwise to ASYNC fixes the rate.

The output control determines the amount of electricity sent to the heart (in milliamperes).

The on-off switch activates the pulse generator.

The battery compartment holds the alkaline batteries.

to function naturally and assist only when necessary. The sensing threshold allows the pacemaker to do this by sensing the heart's normal activity.

SYNCHRONOUS AND ASYNCHRONOUS PACING

Pacemakers can be classified according to sensitivity. In synchronous, or demand, pacing, the pacemaker initiates electrical impulses only when the heart's intrinsic heart rate falls below the preset rate of the pacemaker. In

asynchronous, or fixed, pacing, the pacemaker constantly initiates electrical impulses at a preset rate without regard to the patient's intrinsic electrical activity or heart rate. This type of pacemaker is rarely used.

BIVENTRICULAR PACEMAKERS

The use of a biventricular pacemaker, also referred to as cardiac resynchronization therapy, is being used to treat patients with moderate and severe heart failure who have left ventricular dysynchrony. These patients have intraventricular conduction defects, which result in uncoordinated contraction of the right and left ventricles and a wide QRS complex on an ECG. Left ventricular dysynchrony has been associated with worsening heart failure and increased morbidity and mortality.

Biventricular pacemakers use three leads — one in the right atrium and one in each ventricle — to coordinate ventricular contractions and improve hemodynamic status. Biventricular pacing has been incorporated into certain automatic implantable cardiac defibrillators and has been used as stand-alone therapy.

PACEMAKER DESCRIPTION CODES

The capabilities of pacemakers are described by a five-letter coding system, though three letters are more commonly used. The first letter of the code identifies the heart chambers being paced. Here are the options and the letters used to signify that option:
- V = Ventricle
- A = Atrium
- D = Dual (ventricle and atrium)
- O = None.

The second letter of the code signifies the heart chamber where the pacemaker senses the intrinsic activity. Here are its options:
- V = Ventricle
- A = Atrium
- D = Dual (ventricle and atrium)
- O = None.

The third letter indicates the pacemaker's mode of response to the intrinsic electrical activity it senses in the atrium or ventricle. Its options include:

- T = Triggered pacing. If atrial activity is sensed, for instance, ventricular pacing may be triggered.
- I = Inhibits pacing. If the pacemaker senses intrinsic activity, it won't fire.
- D = Dual. The pacemaker can be triggered or inhibited depending on the mode and where intrinsic activity occurs.
- O = None. The pacemaker doesn't change its mode in response to sensed activity.

The fourth letter of the code describes the pacemaker's programmability. The letter tells whether an external programming device can modify the pacemaker. Here are its options:
- P = Basic functions programmable
- M = Multiprogrammable parameters
- C = Communicating functions such as telemetry
- R = Rate responsiveness or rate modulation, which adjusts to fit the patient's metabolic needs and achieve normal hemodynamic status
- O = None.

The final letter of the code denotes special tachyarrhythmia functions and identifies how the pacemaker responds to a tachyarrhythmia:
- P = Pacing ability. The pacemaker's rapid bursts pace the heart at a rate above its intrinsic rate to override the source of tachycardia. When the stimulation ceases, the tachyarrhythmia breaks. Increased arrhythmia may result.
- S = Shock. An ICD identifies ventricular tachycardia and delivers a shock to stop the arrhythmia.
- D = Dual ability to shock and pace.
- O = None.

AAI and VVI pacemakers

Both an AAI and a VVI pacemaker are single-chamber pacemakers. The electrode for an AAI is placed in the atrium. For a VVI pacemaker, the electrode is placed in the ventricle. These rhythm strips show how each pacemaker works.

AAI pacemaker
Note how the AAI pacemaker senses and paces the atria only. The QRS complex that follows occurs as a result of the heart's own conduction.

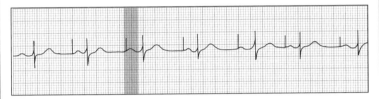

ECG characteristics of AAI pacemakers:

- *P wave:* follows each atrial spike (atrial depolarization) (shaded area)
- *QRS complex:* results from normal conduction

VVI pacemaker
The VVI pacemaker senses and paces the ventricles. When each spike is followed by a depolarization, as shown here, the rhythm is said to reflect 100% capture.

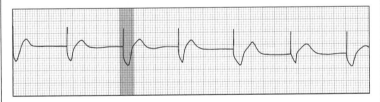

ECG characteristics of VVI pacemakers:

- *QRS complex:* follows each ventricular spike (ventricular depolarization) (shaded area)

PACING MODES
The mode of a pacemaker indicates its functions. Several different modes may be used during pacing, and they may or may not mimic the normal cardiac cycle. A three-letter code, rather than a five-letter code, is typically used to describe pacemaker function. Modes include AAI, VVI, DVI, and DDD. (See *AAI and VVI pacemakers.*)

DVI pacemakers

A committed DVI pacemaker paces the atria and ventricles. The pacemaker senses only ventricular activity. The rhythm strip below shows the effects of a committed DVI pacemaker.

In two of the complexes, the pacemaker didn't sense the intrinsic QRS complex because the complex occurred during the AV interval, when the pacemaker was already committed to fire (shaded areas). With a noncommitted DVI pacemaker, spikes after the QRS complex wouldn't appear because the stimulus to pace the ventricles would be inhibited.

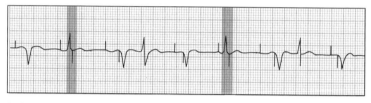

ECG characteristics of committed DVI pacemakers:

• *Ventricular pacemaker:* fires despite the intrinsic QRS complex

AAI mode

The AAI, or atrial demand, pacemaker is a single-chambered pacemaker that paces and senses the atria. When the pacemaker senses intrinsic atrial activity, it inhibits pacing and resets itself. Only the atria are paced.

Because AAI pacemakers require a functioning AV node and intact conduction system, they aren't used in AV block. An AAI pacemaker may be used in patients with sinus bradycardia, which may occur after cardiac surgery, or with sick sinus syndrome, as long as the AV node and His-Purkinje system aren't diseased.

VVI mode

The VVI, or ventricular demand, pacemaker paces and senses the ventricles.

When it senses intrinsic ventricular activity, it inhibits pacing.

This single-chambered pacemaker benefits patients with complete heart block and those needing intermittent pacing. Because it doesn't affect atrial activity, it's used for patients who don't need an atrial kick — the extra 15% to 30% of cardiac output that comes from atrial contraction.

If a patient has spontaneous atrial activity, a VVI pacemaker won't synchronize the ventricular activity with it, so tricuspid and mitral regurgitation may develop. Sedentary patients may receive this pacemaker, but it won't adjust its rate for more active patients.

DVI mode

The DVI, or AV sequential, pacemaker paces the atria and ventricles. (See *DVI*

DDD pacemakers

This rhythm strip shows the effects of a DDD pacemaker. Complexes 1, 2, 4, and 7 reveal the atrial-synchronous mode, set at a rate of 70. The patient has an intrinsic P wave, so the pacemaker serves only to ensure that the ventricles respond.

Complexes 3, 5, 8, 10, and 12 are intrinsic ventricular depolarizations. The pacemaker senses these depolarizations and inhibits firing. In complexes 6, 9, and 11, the pacemaker is pacing the atria and ventricles in sequence. In complex 13, only the atria are paced; the ventricles respond on their own.

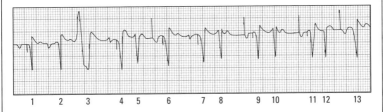

ECG characteristics of DDD pacemakers:

- *1:* pacemaker pacing ventricles only
- *11:* pacemaker pacing atria and ventricles

---

pacemakers.) This dual-chambered pacemaker senses only the ventricles' intrinsic activity, inhibiting ventricular pacing.

Two types of DVI pacemakers may be used, a committed DVI and a non-committed DVI pacemaker. The committed DVI pacemaker doesn't sense intrinsic activity during the AV interval — the time between an atrial and ventricular spike. It generates an impulse even with spontaneous ventricular depolarization. The noncommitted DVI pacemaker, on the other hand, is inhibited if a spontaneous depolarization occurs.

The DVI pacemaker helps patients with AV block or sick sinus syndrome who have a diseased His-Purkinje conduction system. It provides the benefits of AV synchrony and atrial kick, thus improving cardiac output. However, it

can't vary the atrial rate and isn't helpful in atrial fibrillation because it can't capture the atria. In addition, it may needlessly fire or inhibit its own pacing.

DDD mode

A DDD, or universal, pacemaker is used with severe AV block. (See *DDD pacemakers.*) However, because the pacemaker possesses so many capabilities, it may be hard to troubleshoot problems.

Advantages of the DDD pacemaker include its

- versatility
- programmability
- ability to change modes automatically
- ability to mimic the normal physiologic cardiac cycle, maintaining AV synchrony

Evaluating a DDD pacemaker rhythm strip

Look for these potential events when examining a rhythm strip of a patient with a DDD pacemaker.

• Intrinsic rhythm. No pacemaker activity occurs because none is needed.

• Intrinsic P wave followed by a ventricular pacemaker spike. The pacemaker is tracking the atrial rate and assuring a ventricular response.

• Pacemaker spike before a P wave, then an intrinsic ventricular QRS complex. The atrial rate is falling below the lower rate limit, causing the atrial channel to fire. Normal conduction to the ventricles then ensues.

• Pacemaker spike before a P wave and a pacemaker spike before the QRS complex. No intrinsic activity occurs in either the atria or ventricles.

■ ability to sense and pace the atria and ventricles at the same time according to the intrinsic atrial rate and maximal rate limit.

Unlike other pacemakers, the DDD pacemaker is set with a rate range, rather than a single critical rate. It senses atrial activity and ensures that the ventricles respond to each atrial stimulation, thereby maintaining normal AV synchrony.

The DDD pacemaker fires when the ventricle doesn't respond on its own, and it paces the atria when the atrial rate falls below the lower set rate. (See *Evaluating a DDD pacemaker rhythm*

strip.) In a patient with a high atrial rate, a safety mechanism allows the pacemaker to follow the intrinsic atrial rate only to a preset upper limit. That limit is usually set at about 130 beats/minute and helps to prevent the ventricles from responding to atrial tachycardia or atrial flutter.

ASSESSING PACEMAKER FUNCTION

After a pacemaker has been implanted, its function should be assessed. First, determine the pacemaker's mode and settings. If the patient had a permanent pacemaker implanted before admission, ask whether the wallet card from the manufacturer notes the mode and settings.

If the pacemaker was recently implanted, check the patient's medical record for information. Don't check only the ECG tracing — you might misinterpret it if you don't know what kind of pacemaker was used. For instance, if the tracing has ventricular spikes but no atrial pacing spikes, you might assume that it's a VVI pacemaker when it's actually a DVI pacemaker that has lost its atrial output.

Next, review the patient's 12-lead ECG. If it isn't available, examine lead V_1 or MCL_1 instead. Invert the QRS complex here (turn the rhythm strip upside down). An upright QRS complex may mean that the leadwire is out of position, perhaps even perforating the septum and lodging in the left ventricle.

Select a monitoring lead that clearly shows the pacemaker spikes. Make sure the lead you select doesn't cause the cardiac monitor to misinterpret a spike for a QRS complex and double-count the heart rate. This may cause the alarm to sound, falsely signaling a high heart rate.

When looking at an ECG tracing for a patient with a pacemaker, consider the pacemaker mode, and then interpret the paced rhythm. Does it correlate with what you know about the pacemaker?

Look for information that tells you which chamber is paced. Is there capture? Is there a P wave or QRS complex after each atrial or ventricular spike? Or do the P waves and QRS complexes stem from intrinsic electrical activity?

Look for information about the pacemaker's sensing ability. If intrinsic atrial or ventricular activity is present, what is the pacemaker's response?

Look at the rate. What is the pacing rate per minute? Is it appropriate given the pacemaker settings? Although you can determine the rate quickly by counting the number of complexes in a 6-second ECG strip, a more accurate method is to count the number of small boxes between complexes and divide this into 1,500.

Knowing your patient's medical history and whether a pacemaker has been implanted will also help you to determine whether your patient is experiencing ventricular ectopy or paced activity on the ECG. (See *Distinguishing intermittent ventricular pacing from PVCs,* page 162.)

TROUBLESHOOTING PACEMAKER PROBLEMS

A malfunctioning pacemaker can lead to arrhythmias, hypotension, syncope, and other signs and symptoms of decreased cardiac output. (See *Recognizing a malfunctioning pacemaker,* pages 163 and 164.) Common problems with

pacemakers that can lead to low cardiac output and loss of AV synchrony include:
- failure to capture
- failure to pace
- undersensing
- oversensing.

Failure to capture

Failure to capture appears on an ECG as a pacemaker spike without the appropriate atrial or ventricular response — a spike without a complex. Think of failure to capture as the pacemaker's inability to stimulate the chamber.

Causes of failure to capture include acidosis, electrolyte imbalances, fibrosis, incorrect leadwire position, a low milliampere or output setting, depletion of the battery, a broken or cracked leadwire, or perforation of the leadwire through the myocardium.

Failure to pace

Failure to pace is indicated by no pacemaker activity on an ECG when pacemaker activity is appropriately expected. This problem may be caused by battery or circuit failure, cracked or broken leads, or interference between atrial and ventricular sensing in a dual-chambered pacemaker. Failure to pace can lead to asystole.

Undersensing

Undersensing is indicated by a pacemaker spike when intrinsic cardiac activity is already present. In asynchronous pacemakers that have codes, such as VOO or DOO, undersensing is a programming limitation.

When undersensing occurs in synchronous pacemakers, pacing spikes occur on the ECG where they should

Distinguishing intermittent ventricular pacing from PVCs

Knowing whether your patient has an artificial pacemaker will help you avoid mistaking a ventricular paced beat for a premature ventricular contraction (PVC). If your facility uses a monitoring system that eliminates artifact, make sure the monitor is set up correctly for a patient with a pacemaker. Otherwise, the pacemaker spikes may be eliminated as well.

Intermittent ventricular pacing

• The paced ventricular complex will have a pacemaker spike preceding it (shaded area). You may need to look in different leads for a bipolar pacemaker spike because it's small and may be difficult to see.

• The paced ventricular complex of a properly functioning pacemaker won't occur early or prematurely. It will occur only when the patient's own ventricular rate falls below the rate set for the pacemaker.

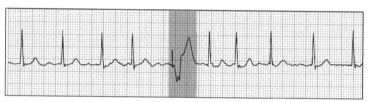

PVC

• PVCs will occur prematurely and won't have pacemaker spikes preceding them (shaded areas).

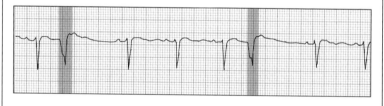

not. Although they may appear in any part of the cardiac cycle, the spikes are especially dangerous if they fall on the T wave, where they can cause ventricular tachycardia or ventricular fibrillation.

In synchronous pacemakers, undersensing may be caused by electrolyte imbalances, disconnection or dislodgment of a lead, improper lead placement, increased sensing threshold from edema or fibrosis at the electrode tip,

TROUBLESHOOTING

Recognizing a malfunctioning pacemaker

Occasionally, pacemakers fail to function properly. When that happens, you'll need to take immediate action to correct the problem. The rhythm strips below show examples of problems that can occur with a temporary pacemaker.

Failure to capture
• If the patient's condition has changed, notify the physician and request new settings.
• If the pacemaker settings have been altered by the patient or someone else, return them to their correct positions. Make sure the face of the pacemaker is covered with its plastic shield. Remind the patient not to touch the dials.
• If the heart still doesn't respond, carefully check all connections. You can also increase the milliampere setting slowly (according to your facility's policy or the physician's orders), turn the patient from side to side, change the battery, and reverse the cables in the pulse generator so the positive wire is in the negative terminal and vice versa. Keep in mind that chest X-rays may be needed to determine electrode position.

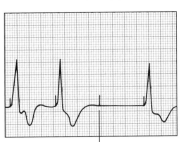

There is a pacemaker spike but no response from the heart.

Failure to pace
• If the pacing or indicator light flashes, check the connections to the cable and the position of the pacing electrode in the patient (performed by X-ray).
• If the pulse generator is turned on but the indicators aren't flashing, change the battery. If the battery is functioning properly, use a different pulse generator.

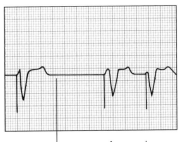

A pacemaker spike should appear here but doesn't.

(continued)

Recognizing a malfunctioning pacemaker (continued)

Failure to sense intrinsic beats

• If the pacemaker is undersensing (it fires but at the wrong times or for the wrong reasons), turn the sensitivity control completely to the right. If the pacemaker is oversensing (it incorrectly senses depolarization and refuses to fire when it should), turn the sensitivity control slightly to the left.

• Change the battery or pulse generator.

• Remove items in the room that might be causing electromechanical interference. Check that the bed is grounded. Unplug each piece of equipment, and then check to see if the interference stops.

• If the pacemaker is still firing on the T wave and all corrective actions have failed, turn off the pacemaker per the physician's order. Make sure atropine is available in case the patient's heart rate drops, and be prepared to initiate cardiopulmonary resuscitation if necessary.

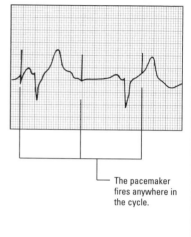

The pacemaker fires anywhere in the cycle.

drug interactions, or a depleted or dead pacemaker battery.

Oversensing

If the pacemaker is too sensitive, it can misinterpret muscle movements or other events in the cardiac cycle as intrinsic cardiac electrical activity. Pacing won't occur when it's needed, and the heart rate and AV synchrony won't be maintained.

INTERVENTIONS

Make sure you're familiar with different types of pacemakers and how they function, so you'll feel more confident in an emergency. When caring for a patient with a pacemaker, follow these guidelines.

▪ Assist with pacemaker insertion as appropriate.

▪ Check the patient's pacemaker settings, connections, and functions regularly.

▪ Monitor the patient to see how well the pacemaker is tolerated.

▪ Reposition a patient who has a temporary pacemaker carefully. Turning may dislodge the leadwire.

▪ Avoid microshocks to the patient by ensuring that the patient's bed and all electrical equipment are grounded properly.

▪ Remember that pacemaker spikes on the monitor don't necessarily mean your patient is stable. Be sure to check the patient's vital signs and assess for signs and symptoms of decreased cardiac output, such as hypotension, chest pain, dyspnea, and syncope.

■ Be alert for signs of infection.

■ Watch for subcutaneous emphysema (air in the subcutaneous tissues) around the pacemaker insertion site. Subcutaneous emphysema feels crunchy under your fingers (crepitus) and may indicate pneumothorax.

■ Look for pectoral muscle twitching or hiccups that occur in synchrony with the pacemaker. Both are signs of abnormal electrical stimulation and possibly perforation. Notify the physician if you note either of these conditions.

■ Watch for signs of a perforated ventricle and the resultant cardiac tamponade. Signs and symptoms include persistent hiccups, tachycardia, distant heart sounds, pulsus paradoxus (a drop in the strength of a pulse during inspiration), hypotension with narrowed pulse pressure, cyanosis, distended neck veins, decreased urine output, restlessness, and complaints of fullness in the chest. Notify the physician immediately if you note any of these signs and symptoms.

PATIENT EDUCATION
Following pacemaker insertion, be sure to cover the following points with the patient and his family:

■ Explain why a pacemaker is needed, how it works, and what can be expected from it.

■ Warn the patient with a temporary pacemaker not to get out of bed without assistance.

■ Warn the patient with a transcutaneous pacemaker to expect twitching of the pectoral muscles. Reassure him that

analgesics will be given if the discomfort becomes intolerable.

■ Instruct the patient not to manipulate the pacemaker wires or pulse generator.

■ Give the patient with a permanent pacemaker the manufacturer's identification card, and tell him that it should be carried at all times.

■ Teach the patient and his family members how to care for the incision, how to take a pulse, and what to do if the pulse drops below the pacemaker rate.

■ Advise the patient to avoid tight clothing or other direct pressure over the pulse generator, to avoid magnetic resonance imaging (MRI) and certain other diagnostic studies, and to notify the physician if confusion, light-headedness, or shortness of breath occur. The patient should also notify the physician if palpitations, hiccups, or a rapid or an unusually slow heart rate occur.

Implantable cardioverter-defibrillators

An ICD is an implanted electronic device that continually monitors the heart for bradycardia, ventricular tachycardia, and ventricular fibrillation (VF). The device then administers either shocks or paced beats to treat the dangerous arrhythmia. In general, ICDs are indicated for patients in whom drug therapy, surgery, or catheter ablation has failed to prevent an arrhythmia.

The system consists of a programmable pulse generator and one or more leadwires. The pulse generator is a

Types of ICD therapies

Implantable cardioverter-defibrillators (ICDs) can deliver a range of therapies, depending on the arrhythmia detected and how the device is programmed. Therapies include antitachycardia pacing, cardioversion, defibrillation, and bradycardia pacing.

Therapy	Description
Antitachycardia pacing	A series of small, rapid electrical pacing pulses used to interrupt ventricular tachycardia (VT) and return the heart to its normal rhythm. Antitachycardia pacing isn't appropriate for all patients and is initiated by the physician after appropriate evaluation of electrophysiology studies.
Cardioversion	A low- or high-energy shock (up to 34 joules) timed to the R wave to terminate VT and return the heart to its normal rhythm.
Defibrillation	A high-energy shock (up to 34 joules) to the heart to terminate ventricular fibrillation and return the heart to its normal rhythm.
Bradycardia pacing	Electrical pacing pulses used when the natural electrical signals are too slow. Most ICD systems can pace one chamber (VVI pacing) of the heart at a preset rate. Some systems will sense and pace both chambers (DDD pacing).

small computer powered by a battery that's responsible for monitoring the heart's electrical activity and delivering electrical therapy when it identifies an abnormal rhythm.

It also stores information on the heart's electrical activity before, during, and after an arrhythmia, along with tracking which treatment was delivered and the outcome of that treatment. Many devices store electrograms (electrical tracings similar to ECGs). With an interrogation device, a physician can retrieve this information, evaluate ICD function and battery status, and adjust ICD system settings when indicated.

The leads are insulated wires that carry cardiac electrical signals to the pulse generator and deliver electrical energy from the pulse generator to the heart.

Today's advanced devices can detect a wide range of arrhythmias and automatically respond with the appropriate therapy, such as bradycardia pacing (both single- and dual-chamber), antitachycardia pacing, cardioversion, and defibrillation. ICDs that provide therapy for atrial arrhythmias, such as atrial fibrillation, are under evaluation. (See *Types of ICD therapies*.)

PROCEDURE

ICD implantation is commonly performed in the cardiac catheterization laboratory by a specially trained cardiologist. Occasionally, a patient who requires other cardiac surgery may have the device implanted in the operating room. (See *Location of an ICD*.)

COMPLICATIONS

Complications of ICD implantation include serous or bloody drainage from the insertion site, swelling, ecchymosis, incisional pain, and impaired mobility. Other complications include venous thrombosis, embolism, infection, pneumothorax, pectoral or diaphragmatic muscle stimulation from the ICD, arrhythmias, cardiac tamponade, heart failure, and abnormal ICD operation with lead dislodgment. Failure to function is a late complication and may result in untreated VF and cardiac arrest.

INTERVENTIONS

When caring for a patient with an ICD, know how the device is programmed. This information is available through a status report that can be obtained and printed when the physician or trained technician interrogates the device. This involves placing a specialized piece of equipment over the implanted pulse generator to retrieve pacing function. Program information includes:
- type and model of ICD
- status of the device (on or off)
- detection rates
- therapies that will be delivered, such as pacing, antitachycardia pacing, cardioversion, and defibrillation.

If the patient experiences an arrhythmia or if the device delivers a therapy, this information helps in the evaluation of functioning. (See *Analyzing ICD function*, page 168.)
- If cardiac arrest occurs, initiate cardiopulmonary resuscitation (CPR) and advanced cardiac life support.

Location of an ICD

To insert an implantable cardioverter-defibrillator (ICD), the cardiologist makes a small incision near the clavicle and gains access to the subclavian vein. The lead-wires are inserted through the subclavian vein, threaded into the heart, and placed in contact with the endocardium.

The leads are connected to the pulse generator, which is inserted under the skin in a specially prepared pocket in the right or left upper chest. (Placement is similar to that used for a pacemaker.) The incision is then closed and the device programmed.

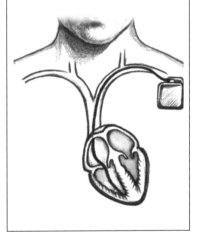

- If the ICD delivers a shock while you're performing chest compressions, you may feel a slight shock. Wearing latex gloves can eliminate this risk.
- It's safe to externally defibrillate the patient as long as the paddles aren't placed directly over the pulse generator. The anteroposterior paddle position is preferred.

Analyzing ICD function

To evaluate the function of an implantable cardioverter-defibrillator (ICD), compare the monitor strips with the device status report. The example shown here demonstrates proper device functioning for ventricular tachycardia (VT) according to the programmed parameters. When VT occurs, the device is programmed to deliver antitachycardia pacing consisting of eight pacing stimuli six separate times. If the arrhythmia doesn't terminate or deteriorates to ventricular fibrillation, the device is programmed to deliver a cardioversion shock. This episode of VT converts to normal sinus rhythm with the first cardioversion.

Status report

VT therapy	1	2	3	4
Therapy status	On	On	On	On
Therapy type	ATP	CV	CV	CV
Initial # pulses	8			
# Sequences	6			
Energy (J)		10	34	34
Waveform		Biphasic	Biphasic	Biphasic

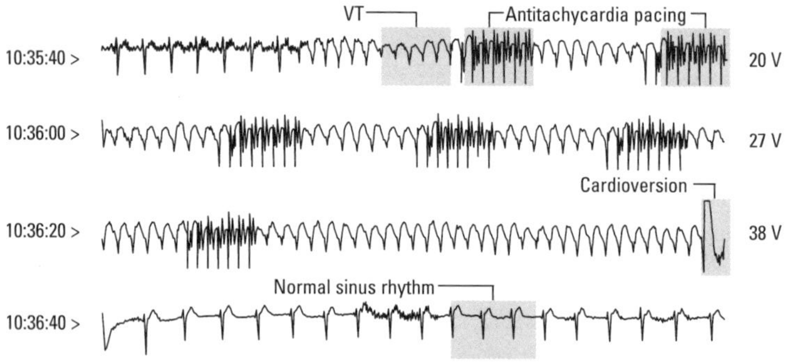

- Be on guard for signs of a perforated ventricle, with resultant cardiac tamponade. Ominous signs include persistent hiccups, distant heart sounds, pulsus paradoxus, hypotension accompanied by narrow pulse pressure, increased venous pressure, distended neck veins, cyanosis, restlessness, and complaints of fullness in the chest. Report any of these signs immediately and prepare the patient for possible emergency surgery.
- Assess the area around the incision for swelling, tenderness, and hema-

Left ventricular assist device

Ventricular assist devices (VADs) are commonly used as a bridge to heart transplantation. A completely implanted left VAD is illustrated below.

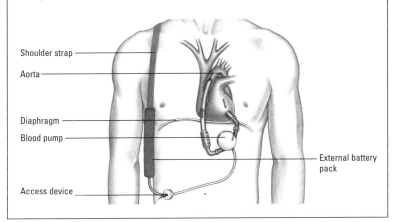

toma, but don't remove the occlusive dressing for the first 24 hours without a physician's order. When you remove the dressing, check the wound for drainage, redness, and unusual warmth or tenderness.

■ After the first 24 hours, begin passive range-of-motion exercises if ordered, and progress as tolerated.

PATIENT EDUCATION

■ Tell the patient to wear medical identification indicating ICD placement.
■ Educate family members in emergency techniques, such as activating the local emergency medical system and performing CPR, in case the device fails.
■ Warn the patient to avoid placing excessive pressure over the insertion site or moving or jerking the area until after the postoperative visit.
■ Tell the patient to follow normal routines as allowed by the physician and to increase exercise as tolerated.

■ Remind the patient to carry information regarding his ICD at all times and to inform the appropriate personnel when traveling or undergoing diagnostic procedures, such as computed tomography scans or MRI.
■ Explain that electronic devices may cause disruption of the ICD.
■ Stress the importance of follow-up care and physician checkups.

Ventricular assist devices

VADs are designed to decrease the heart's workload and increase cardiac output in patients with ventricular failure. Left ventricular, right ventricular, and biventricular VADs are available. (See *Left ventricular assist device.*)

Understanding orthotopic heart transplantation

The illustration below shows how the donor heart is anastomosed to the recipient's right atrium.

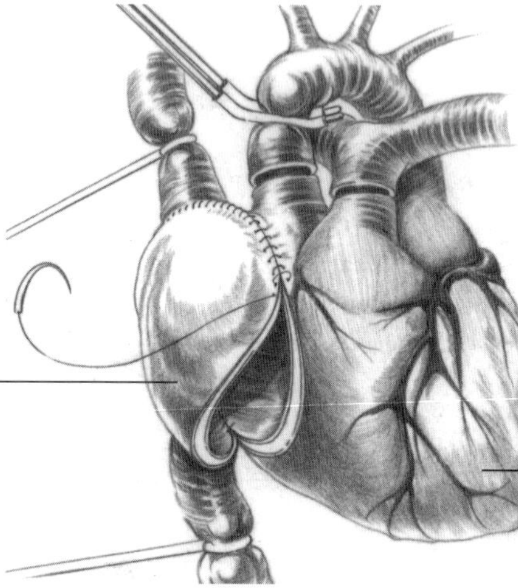

Recipient's right atrial wall

Donor heart

In a surgical procedure, blood is diverted from a ventricle to an artificial pump, which maintains systemic perfusion. VADs are commonly used as a bridge to maintain perfusion until a heart transplantation procedure can be performed.

VADs may be indicated for patients who can't be weaned from cardiopulmonary bypass (CPB) or intra-aortic balloon pump as well as for those patients who are awaiting heart transplantation.

Because a VAD supports the heart's pumping function rather than altering electrical function, it doesn't affect the heart's electrical activity. As a result, you probably won't see ECG changes caused by the VAD. However, studies currently being conducted are evaluating possible changes in the ECG of patients following the implantation of a VAD.

Heart transplantation

Some patients with end-stage cardiac disease may be candidates for heart transplantation. Two types of heart transplantation may be performed: orthotopic and heterotopic.

ORTHOTOPIC HEART TRANSPLANTATION

Orthotopic heart transplantation (OHT) is the most commonly performed procedure. OHT involves removal of most of the patient's heart (native heart), retaining a large portion of the right and left atria.

OHT involves a median sternotomy and use of CPB. The donor heart is attached (anastomosed) to the native atrial cusps, and direct end-to-end anastomoses of the aorta and pulmonary artery are performed. (See *Understanding orthotopic heart transplantation.*)

In OHT, the transplanted heart is denervated so it can't respond normally to stimuli from the autonomic nervous system. Initially, electrical activity in the new heart is slow, requiring the use of a temporary pacemaker in the immediate postoperative period. Bradycardia due to chronotropic incompetence may occur as a result of either primary sinus node dysfunction or the use of preoperative negative chronotropic agents such as amiodarone.

The denervated transplanted heart also has a blunted response to exercise. That's because the transplanted heart relies on circulating catecholamines to respond to the demands of an increased heart rate. Although there have been reports of reinnervation of the recipient heart 1 year posttransplant, the response to exercise is generally considered diminished in all cases.

It's important to remember that in OHT, the sinus node of the native heart remains intact. This accounts for the two P waves frequently seen on the posttransplant ECG. (See *ECG waveform after orthotopic heart transplantation.*) However, only the sinus node of the donor heart conducts through to the ventricles.

ECG waveform after orthotopic heart transplantation

An orthotopic heart transplantation leads to characteristic findings on an electrocardiogram (ECG). For example, the waveform below shows two distinct types of P waves. P waves caused by the native heart's SA node are unrelated to the QRS complexes (first shaded area). P waves caused by the donor heart's SA node precede each QRS complex (second shaded area).

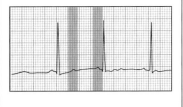

Abnormalities of the donor SA node's conduction and automaticity frequently occur as a result of injury to the donor heart during procurement, transportation, or transplantation. If the conduction system is damaged or if the SA node fails to function properly after the heart is transplanted, the ECG will reflect the abnormality.

Following heart transplantation, supraventricular and ventricular arrhythmias as well as ventricular conduction defects are common. Atrial fibrillation and other arrhythmias can signal acute rejection.

ECG characteristics

Rate: Atrial and ventricular rates are frequently slow, requiring the use of a

ECG waveform after heterotopic heart transplantation

This strip shows the ECG of the recipient's own heart (first shaded area) and the donor heart (second shaded area).

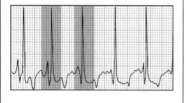

temporary pacemaker in the immediate postoperative period or therapy with drugs such as theophylline.

Rhythm: The patient's native P waves will have a regular rhythm unrelated to the QRS complexes of the donor heart. The donor atrial and ventricular rhythms are usually regular.

P waves: Two separate P waves are typically seen: the P wave of the donor heart and the P wave of the native heart.

QRS complex: May be widened secondary to ventricular conduction defects.

Other: Pacemaker activity should appear as long as the patient requires pacemaker support for chronotropic incompetence.

HETEROTOPIC HEART TRANSPLANTATION

Heterotopic heart transplantation, less commonly performed, involves graft-ing a donor heart to a recipient heart, without removing the recipient heart. The donor heart is used to assist the pumping ability of the native heart. This procedure is also referred to as "piggyback" heart transplantation.

ECG characteristics

Because a heterotopic heart transplantation provides the patient with a second functioning heart, the ECG shows two distinct cardiac rhythms. You can usually differentiate the native rhythm from the donor rhythm by analyzing the recipient's preoperative ECG. In addition, the QRS complex of the donor heart frequently has a greater amplitude. (See *ECG waveform after heterotopic heart transplantation.*)

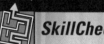

SkillCheck

1. Which of the following electrolyte disturbances commonly causes classic tall, peaked T waves on an ECG?
   a. Hypokalemia
   b. Hypocalcemia
   c. Hypercalcemia
   d. Hyperkalemia

Answer: d. The presence of tall, peaked T waves is characteristic of hyperkalemia.

2. Which of the following categories of antiarrhythmic drugs is also known as sodium channel drugs?
   a. Class I
   b. Class II
   c. Class III
   d. Class IV

Answer: a. Class I drugs block the

influx of sodium into the cell during phase 0 of the action potential, also referred to as the sodium channel or fast channel. Thus, these drugs may also be called sodium channel blockers or fast channel blockers.

3. The following ECG strip shows the characteristic effect of which of the following cardiac drugs?
  a. procainamide
  b. flecainide
  c. quinidine
  d. digoxin

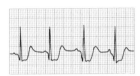

Answer: d. Digoxin, the most commonly used cardiac glycoside, typically causes a characteristic sagging of the ST segment.

4. The ECG below shows which of the following pacemaker problems?
  a. Failure to pace
  b. Undersensing
  c. Failure to capture
  d. Oversensing

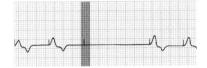

Answer: c. Failure to capture is characterized by appropriately appearing pacemaker spikes on the ECG not followed by P waves or QRS complexes (depending on the chamber or chambers to be paced).

5. Which of the following procedures causes the characteristic ECG changes on the rhythm strip below?
  a. Implantable cardioverter-defibrillator (ICD)
  b. Orthotopic heart transplant (OHT)
  c. Ventricular assist device (VAD)
  d. Heterotopic heart transplant

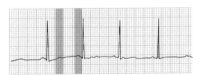

Answer: b. The waveform shows an ECG from a patient with an OHT. There are two kinds of P waves present: one initiated by the patient's own SA node, which is unrelated to the QRS complex, and one initiated by the donor SA node, which precedes each QRS complex.

The 12-lead electrocardiogram (ECG) is a diagnostic test that helps identify pathologic conditions, especially angina and acute myocardial infarction (MI). It provides a more complete view of the heart's electrical activity than a rhythm strip and can be used to assess left ventricular function more effectively. Patients with conditions that affect the heart's electrical system may also benefit from a 12-lead ECG, including those with:

- cardiac arrhythmias
- heart chamber enlargement or hypertrophy
- digoxin or other drug toxicity
- electrolyte imbalances
- pulmonary embolism
- pericarditis
- pacemakers
- hypothermia.

Like other diagnostic tests, a 12-lead ECG must be viewed in conjunction with other clinical data. Therefore, always correlate the patient's ECG results with the history, physical assessment findings, and results of laboratory and other diagnostic studies as well as the drug regimen.

Remember, too, that an ECG can be done in a variety of ways, including over a telephone line. (See *Transtelephonic cardiac monitoring*.) In fact, transtelephonic monitoring has become increasingly important as a tool for assessing patients at home and in other nonclinical settings.

The 12-lead ECG records the heart's electrical activity using a series of electrodes placed on the patient's extremities and chest wall. The 12 leads include three bipolar limb leads (I, II, III), three unipolar augmented limb leads (aV_R, aV_L, and aV_F), and six unipolar precordial, or chest, leads (V_1, V_2, V_3, V_4, V_5, and V_6). These leads provide 12 different views of the heart's electrical activity. (See *ECG leads,* page 176.)

Scanning up, down, and across, each lead transmits information about a different area of the heart. The waveforms obtained from each lead vary depending on the location of the lead in relation to the wave of depolarization passing through the myocardium.

Limb leads

The six limb leads record electrical activity in the heart's frontal plane, a view through the middle of the heart from top to bottom. Electrical activity is recorded from the anterior to the posterior axes.

Transtelephonic cardiac monitoring

Using a special recorder-transmitter, patients at home can transmit ECGs by telephone to a central monitoring center for immediate interpretation. This technique, called transtelephonic cardiac monitoring (TTM), reduces health care costs and is being used more often.

Nurses play an important role in TTM. Besides performing extensive patient and family teaching, they may operate the central monitoring center and help interpret ECGs sent by patients.

TTM allows a health care professional to assess transient conditions that cause such symptoms as palpitations, dizziness, syncope, confusion, paroxysmal dyspnea, and chest pain. Such conditions, which are commonly not apparent while the patient is with a health care professional, can make diagnosis difficult and costly.

With TTM, the patient can transmit an ECG recording from his home when the symptoms appear, avoiding the need to go to the hospital and offering a greater opportunity for early diagnosis. Even if symptoms seldom appear, the patient can keep the equipment for long periods, which further aids in the diagnosis of the patient's condition.

Home care
TTM can also be used by a patient having cardiac rehabilitation at home. He'll be called regularly during this period to assess his progress. Because of this continuous monitoring, TTM can help reduce the anxiety felt by the patient and his family after discharge, especially if the patient suffered a myocardial infarction.

TTM is especially valuable for assessing the effects of drugs and for diagnosing and managing paroxysmal arrhythmias. In both cases, TTM can eliminate the need for admitting the patient for evaluation and a potentially lengthy hospital stay.

Understanding TTM equipment
TTM requires three main pieces of equipment: an ECG recorder-transmitter, a standard telephone line, and a receiver. The ECG recorder-transmitter converts electrical activity from the patient's heart into acoustic waves. Some models contain built-in memory devices that store recordings of cardiac activity for transmission later.

A standard telephone line is used to transmit information. The receiver converts the acoustic waves transmitted over the telephone line into ECG activity, which is then recorded on ECG paper for interpretation and documentation in the patient's chart. The recorder-transmitter uses two types of electrodes applied to the finger and chest. The electrodes produce ECG tracings similar to those of a standard 12-lead ECG.

Credit card-size recorder
One recently developed recorder operates on a battery and is about the size of a credit card. When a patient becomes symptomatic, he holds the back of the card firmly to the center of his chest and pushes the start button. Four electrodes located on the back of the card sense electrical activity and record it. The card can store 30 seconds of activity and can later transmit the recording across phone lines for evaluation by a clinician.

ECG leads

Each of the leads on a 12-lead ECG views the heart from a different angle. These illustrations show the direction of electrical activity (depolarization) monitored by each lead and the 12 views of the heart.

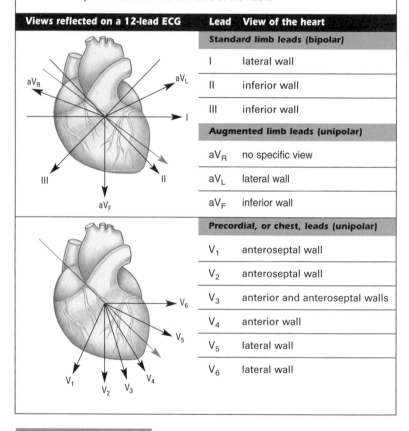

Views reflected on a 12-lead ECG	Lead	View of the heart
	Standard limb leads (bipolar)	
	I	lateral wall
	II	inferior wall
	III	inferior wall
	Augmented limb leads (unipolar)	
	aV_R	no specific view
	aV_L	lateral wall
	aV_F	inferior wall
	Precordial, or chest, leads (unipolar)	
	V_1	anteroseptal wall
	V_2	anteroseptal wall
	V_3	anterior and anteroseptal walls
	V_4	anterior wall
	V_5	lateral wall
	V_6	lateral wall

Precordial leads

The six precordial leads provide information on electrical activity in the heart's horizontal plane, a transverse view through the middle of the heart, dividing it into upper and lower portions. Electrical activity is recorded from either a superior or an inferior approach.

Electrical axes

Besides assessing 12 different leads, a 12-lead ECG records the heart's electrical axis. The term axis refers to the direction of depolarization as it spreads through the heart. As impulses travel through the heart, they generate small electrical forces called instantaneous vectors. The mean of these vectors represents the force and direction of the wave of depolarization through the heart—the electrical axis. The electrical axis is also called the mean instantaneous vector and the mean QRS vector.

In a healthy heart, impulses originate in the sinoatrial (SA) node, travel through the atria to the atrioventricular (AV) node, and then to the ventricles. Most of the movement of the impulses is downward and to the left, the direction of a normal axis.

In an unhealthy heart, axis direction varies. That's because the direction of electrical activity travels away from areas of damage or necrosis and toward areas of hypertrophy. Knowing the normal deflection of each lead will help you evaluate whether the electrical axis is normal or abnormal.

Obtaining a 12-lead ECG

To perform a 12-lead ECG, you'll need to prepare properly, select the appropriate electrode sites, understand how to perform variations on a standard 12-lead ECG, and make an accurate recording.

PREPARATION

Gather all necessary supplies, including the ECG machine, recording paper, electrodes, and gauze pads. Tell the patient that the physician has ordered an ECG, and explain the procedure. Emphasize that the test takes about 10 minutes and that it's a safe and painless way to evaluate the heart's electrical activity. Answer the patient's questions, and offer reassurance. Preparing the patient properly will help alleviate anxiety and promote cooperation.

Ask the patient to lie in a supine position in the center of the bed with arms at the sides. If he can't tolerate lying flat, raise the head of the bed to semi-Fowler's position. Ensure privacy, and expose the patient's arms, legs, and chest, draping for comfort.

SITE SELECTION

Select the areas where you'll apply the electrodes. Choose areas that are flat and fleshy and not muscular or bony. Shave the area if it's excessively hairy. Remove excess oil and other substances from the skin to enhance electrode contact. Remember, the better the electrode contact, the better the recording.

The 12-lead ECG provides 12 different views of the heart, just as 12 photographers snapping the same picture would produce 12 different photographs. Taking all of those snapshots requires placing four electrodes on the limbs and six across the front of the chest wall.

To help ensure an accurate recording, the electrodes must be applied correctly. Inaccurate placement of an electrode by greater than $\frac{3}{5}''$ (1.5 cm) from its standardized position may lead to inaccurate waveforms and an incorrect ECG interpretation.

Limb lead placement

To record the bipolar limb leads I, II, and III and the unipolar limb leads

Limb lead placement

Proper lead placement is critical for the accurate recording of cardiac rhythms. The diagrams here show electrode placement for the six limb leads. RA indicates right arm; LA, left arm; RL, right leg; and LL, left leg. The plus sign (+) indicates the positive pole, the minus sign (–) indicates the negative pole, and G indicates the ground. Below each diagram is a sample ECG recording for that lead.

Lead I
This lead connects the right arm (negative pole) with the left arm (positive pole).

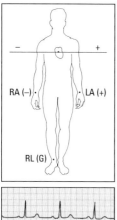

Lead II
This lead connects the right arm (negative pole) with the left leg (positive pole).

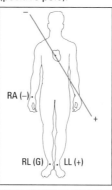
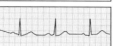

Lead III
This lead connects the left arm (negative pole) with the left leg (positive pole).

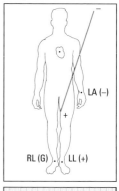
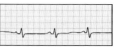

aV_R, aV_L, and aV_F, place electrodes on both of the patient's arms and on his left leg. The right leg also receives an electrode, but that electrode acts as a ground and doesn't contribute to the waveform. (See *Limb lead placement.*)

Placing the electrodes on the patient is typically easy because each leadwire is labeled or color-coded. For example, a wire (usually white) might be labeled "RA" for right arm. Another (usually red) might be labeled "LL" for left leg.

Precordial lead placement
Precordial leads are also labeled or color-coded according to which wire corresponds to which lead. To record the six precordial leads (V_1 through V_6), position the electrodes on specific areas of the anterior chest wall. (See *Precordial lead placement,* page 180.) If they're placed too low, the ECG tracing will be inaccurate.

■ Place lead V_1 over the fourth intercostal space at the right sternal border.

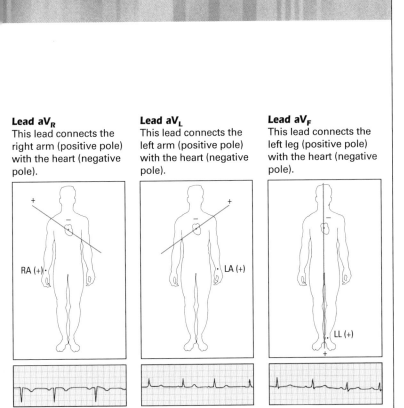

Lead aV_R
This lead connects the right arm (positive pole) with the heart (negative pole).

Lead aV_L
This lead connects the left arm (positive pole) with the heart (negative pole).

Lead aV_F
This lead connects the left leg (positive pole) with the heart (negative pole).

To find the space, locate the sternal notch at the second rib and feel your way down the sternal border until you reach the fourth intercostal space.

■ Place lead V_2 just opposite V_1, over the fourth intercostal space at the left sternal border.

■ Place lead V_4 over the fifth intercostal space at the left midclavicular line. Placing lead V_4 before V_3 makes it easier to see where to place lead V_3.

■ Place lead V_3 midway between V_2 and V_4.

■ Place lead V_5 over the fifth intercostal space at the left anterior axillary line.

■ Place lead V_6 over the fifth intercostal space at the left midaxillary line. If you've placed leads V_4 through V_6 correctly, they should line up horizontally.

Additional types of ECGs

In addition to the standard 12-lead ECG, two other types of ECGs may be used for diagnostic purposes: the posterior-lead ECG and the right chest lead

Precordial lead placement

The precordial leads complement the limb leads to provide a complete view of the heart. To record the precordial leads, place the electrodes as shown.

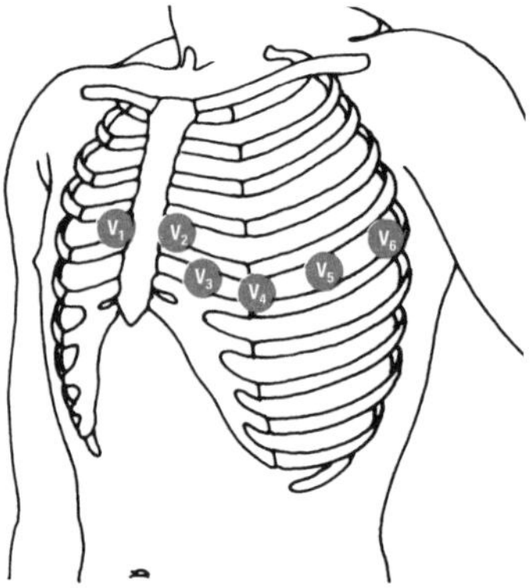

V₁

V₂

V₃

V₄

V₅

V₆

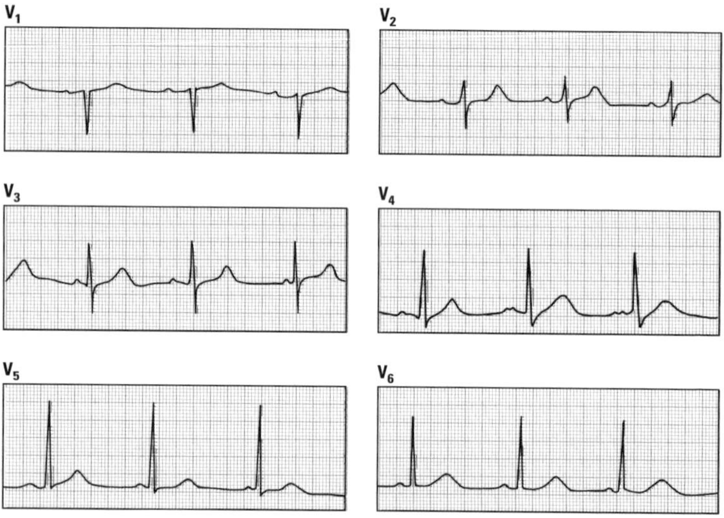

ECG. These ECGs use chest leads to assess areas that standard 12-lead ECGs can't.

POSTERIOR-LEAD ECG

Because of lung and muscle barriers, the usual chest leads can't "see" the heart's posterior surface to record myo-cardial damage there. So some physicians add three posterior leads to the 12-lead ECG: leads V_7, V_8, and V_9. These leads are placed opposite anterior leads V_4, V_5, and V_6, on the left side of the patient's back, following the same horizontal line, as shown at top of next page.

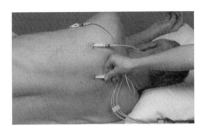

Occasionally, a physician may request right-sided posterior leads. These leads are labeled V_{7R}, V_{8R}, and V_{9R} and are placed on the right side of the patient's back. Their placement is a mirror image of the electrodes on the left side of the back. This type of ECG provides information on the right posterior area of the heart.

RIGHT CHEST LEAD ECG

The standard 12-lead ECG evaluates only the left ventricle. If the right ventricle needs to be assessed for damage or dysfunction, the physician may order a right chest lead ECG. For example, a patient with an inferior wall MI might have a right chest lead ECG to rule out right ventricular involvement.

With this type of ECG, the six leads are placed on the right side of the chest in a mirror image of the standard precordial lead placement, as shown below. Electrodes start at the left sternal border and swing down under the right breast area.

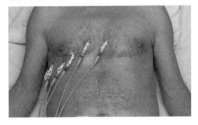

RECORDING THE ECG

After properly placing the electrodes, record the ECG. ECG machines come in two types: multichannel recorders and single-channel recorders. With a multichannel recorder, all electrodes are attached to the patient at once and the machine prints a simultaneous view of all leads. With a single-channel recorder, one lead at a time is recorded in a short strip by attaching and removing electrodes and stopping and starting the tracing each time.

To record an ECG, follow these steps:

- Plug the cord of the ECG machine into a grounded outlet. If the machine operates on a charged battery, it may not need to be plugged in.
- Place one or all of the electrodes on the patient's chest, based on the type of machine you're using.
- Make sure all leads are securely attached, and then turn on the machine.
- Instruct the patient to relax, lie still, and breathe normally. Ask him not to talk during the recording, to prevent distortion of the ECG tracing.
- Set the ECG paper speed selector to 25 mm per second. If necessary, enter the patient's identification data. Then calibrate or standardize the machine according to the manufacturer's instructions.
- Press the AUTO button and record the ECG. For a right chest lead ECG, press the appropriate button for recording.
- Observe the quality of the tracing. When the machine finishes the recording, turn it off.
- Remove the electrodes, and clean the patient's skin.

Multichannel ECG recording

The top of a 12-lead ECG recording usually shows patient identification information along with an interpretation by the machine. A rhythm strip is commonly included at the bottom of the recording.

Standardization

Look for standardization marks on the recording, normally 10 small squares high. If the patient has high voltage complexes, the marks will be half as high. You'll also notice that lead markers separate the lead recordings on the paper and that each lead is labeled.

Familiarize yourself with the order in which the leads are arranged on an ECG tracing. Getting accustomed to the layout of the tracing will help you interpret the ECG more quickly and accurately.

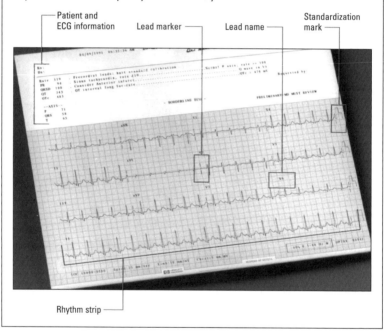

ECG RECORDING

ECG tracings from multichannel and single-channel machines look the same. (See *Multichannel ECG recording*.) The printout will show the patient's name and room number and, possibly, his medical record number. At the top of the printout, you'll see the patient's heart rate and wave durations, measured in seconds.

Some machines are capable of recording ST-segment elevation and depression. The name of the lead will appear next to each 6-second strip.

Be sure to write the following information on the printout: date, time, phy-

Electrode placement for a signal-averaged ECG

Positioning electrodes for a signal-averaged ECG is much different than for a 12-lead ECG. Here's one method:

1. Place the positive X electrode at the left fourth intercostal space, midaxillary line.
2. Place the negative X electrode at the right fourth intercostal space, midaxillary line.
3. Place the positive Y electrode at the left iliac crest.
4. Place the negative Y electrode at the superior aspect of the manubrium of the sternum.
5. Place the positive Z electrode at the fourth intercostal space, left of the sternum.
6. Place the ground (G) on the lower right at the eighth rib.
7. Reposition the patient on his side, or have him sit forward. Then place the negative Z electrode on his back (not shown), directly posterior to the positive Z electrode.
8. Attach all the leads to the electrodes, being careful not to dislodge the posterior lead. Now, you can obtain the tracing.

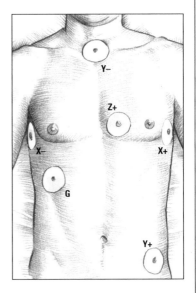

sician's name, and special circumstances. For example, you might record an episode of chest pain, abnormal electrolyte levels, related drug treatment, abnormal placement of the electrodes, or the presence of an artificial pacemaker and whether or not a magnet was used while the ECG was obtained.

Remember, ECGs are legal documents. They belong in the patient's medical record and must be saved for future reference and comparison with baseline strips.

Signal-averaged ECG

Although a standard 12-lead ECG is obtained on most patients, some may benefit from obtaining a signal-averaged ECG. This simple, noninvasive test helps identify patients at risk for sudden death from sustained ventricular tachycardia.

The test uses a computer to identify late electrical potentials — tiny impulses that follow normal depolarization. A standard 12-lead ECG can't detect late electrical potentials. Patients prone to ventricular tachycardia — those who have had a recent MI or unexplained syncope, for example — are good candidates for a signal-averaged ECG. Keep in mind that 12-lead ECGs should be done when the patient is free from arrhythmias.

A signal-averaged ECG is a noise-free, surface ECG recording taken from three specialized leads for several hundred heartbeats. (See *Electrode placement for a signal-averaged ECG,* page 183.) The test takes approximately 10 minutes. The machine's computer detects late electrical potentials and then enlarges them so they're recognizable. The electrodes for a signal-averaged ECG are labeled X–, X+, Y–, Y+, Z–, Z+, and ground.

The machine averages signals from these leads to produce one representative QRS complex without artifact. The process cancels out noise, electrical impulses that don't occur as a repetitious pattern or with the same consistent timing as the QRS complex. With noise filtered out, late electrical potentials can be detected. Muscle noise can't be filtered, however, so the patient must lie still for the test.

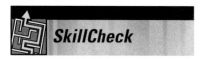

SkillCheck

1. Which of the following limb leads connects the left leg (positive pole) with the heart (negative pole)?
  a. I
  b. III
  c. aV_L
  d. aV_F

Answer: d. Lead aV_F connects the left leg (positive pole) with the heart (negative pole).

2. Which of the following lead placements is the correct one for the precordial lead V_6?
  a. Fourth intercostal space at the right sternal border
  b. Fifth intercostal space at the left midclavicular line
  c. Fifth intercostal space at the left anterior axillary line
  d. Fifth intercostal space at the left midaxillary line

Answer: d. Lead V_6 is placed over the fifth intercostal space at the left midaxillary line.

3. Which of the following types of ECG uses a computer to identify late electrical potentials?
  a. Signal-averaged
  b. Standard 12-lead
  c. Right chest lead
  d. Posterior lead

Answer: a. A signal-averaged ECG uses a computer to identify late electrical potentials, helping to identify patients at risk for sudden death from sustained ventricular tachycardia.

4. Leads II, III, and aV_F look at which of the following views of the heart?
  a. Lateral wall
  b. Inferior wall
  c. Anterior wall
  d. Anteroseptal wall

Answer: b. Leads II, III, and aV_F look at the inferior wall of the heart.

5. If your patient's ECG showed ST-segment elevation in leads I, aV_L, V_5, and V_6, you would be concerned that he was experiencing which of the following types of MI?

a. Anterior wall
b. Inferior wall
c. Lateral wall
d. Right ventricular wall

Answer: c. Leads I, aV_L, V_5, and V_6 look at the lateral wall of the heart and so would indicate a lateral wall MI.

With an electrocardiogram (ECG) in hand, the final skill involves interpreting the rhythm and understanding how various disorders can affect those interpretations. This chapter examines ECG interpretation and variations in such disorders as angina, bundle-branch block, myocardial infarction (MI), pericarditis, Prinzmetal's variant angina, and left ventricular hypertrophy.

Interpreting ECGs

To interpret a 12-lead ECG, use a systematic approach. Compare the patient's previous ECG with the current one, if available. This will help you identify changes.

Steps in interpretation

1. Check the ECG tracing to see if it's technically correct. Make sure the baseline is free from electrical interference and drift.
2. Scan the limb leads I, II, and III. The R-wave voltage in lead II should equal the sum of the R-wave voltage in leads I and III. Lead aV_R is typically negative. If these rules aren't met, the tracing may be recorded incorrectly.
3. Locate the lead markers on the

waveform. Lead markers are the points where one lead changes to another.
4. Check the standardization markings to make sure all leads were recorded with the ECG machine's amplitude at the same setting. Standardization markings are usually located at the beginning of the strip.
5. Assess the heart's rate and rhythm.
6. Determine the heart's electrical axis. Use either the quadrant method or the degree method, which are described later in this chapter.
7. Examine limb leads I, II, and III. The R wave in lead II should be taller than in lead I. The R wave in lead III should be a smaller version of the R wave in lead I. The P wave or QRS complex may be inverted. Each lead should have flat ST segments and upright T waves. Pathologic Q waves should be absent.
8. Examine limb leads aV_L, aV_F, and aV_R. The tracings from leads aV_L and aV_F should be similar, but lead aV_F should have taller P and R waves. Lead aV_R has little diagnostic value. Its P wave, QRS complex, and T wave should be deflected downward.
9. Examine the R wave in the precordial leads. Normally, the R wave — the first positive deflection of the QRS complex — gets progressively taller from lead V_1 to V_5. It gets slightly smaller in lead V_6. (See *R-wave progression.*)
10. Examine the S wave (the negative

deflection after an R wave) in the precordial leads. It should appear extremely deep in lead V_1 and become progressively more shallow, usually disappearing by lead V_5.

Waveform abnormalities

As you examine each lead, note where changes occur so you can identify the area of the heart affected. Remember that P waves should be upright; however, they may be inverted in lead aV_R or biphasic or inverted in leads III, aV_L, and V_1.

PR intervals should always be constant, just like QRS-complex durations. QRS-complex deflections will vary in different leads. Observe for pathologic Q waves.

ST segments should be isoelectric or have minimal deviation. ST-segment elevation greater than 1 mm above the baseline and ST-segment depression greater than 0.5 mm below the baseline are considered abnormal. Leads facing an injured area will have ST-segment elevations, and leads facing away will show ST-segment depressions.

The T wave normally deflects upward in leads I, II, and V_3 through V_6. It's inverted in lead aV_R and variable in the other leads. T-wave changes have many causes and aren't always a reason for alarm. Excessively tall, flat, or inverted T waves occurring with symptoms, such as chest pain, may indicate ischemia.

A normal Q wave generally has a duration of under 0.04 second. An abnormal Q wave has either a duration of

R-wave progression

R waves should progress normally through the precordial leads. Note that the R wave in this strip is the first positive deflection in the QRS complex. Also note that the S wave gets smaller, or regresses, from lead V_1 to V_6 until it finally disappears.

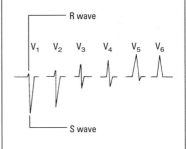

0.04 second or more, a depth greater than 4 mm, or a height one-fourth of the R wave.

Abnormal Q waves indicate myocardial necrosis. These waves develop when depolarization can't follow its normal path due to damaged tissue in the area. Lead aV_R normally has a large Q wave, so disregard this lead when searching for abnormal Q waves.

Electrical axis

The electrical axis is the average direction of the heart's electrical activity during ventricular depolarization. Leads placed on the body sense the sum of the heart's electrical activity and record it as waveforms.

You can determine your patient's electrical axis by examining the wave-

Hexaxial reference system

The hexaxial reference system consists of six bisecting lines, each representing one of the six limb leads, and a circle, representing the heart. The intersection of all lines divides the circle into equal, 30-degree segments.

Shifting degrees

Note that 0 degrees appears at the 3 o'clock position (positive pole lead I). Moving counterclockwise, the degrees become increasingly negative, until reaching ± 180 degrees, at the 9 o'clock position (negative pole lead I).

The bottom half of the circle contains the corresponding positive degrees. However, a positive-degree designation doesn't necessarily mean that the pole is positive.

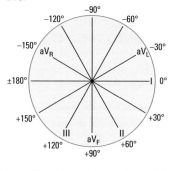

forms recorded from the six frontal plane leads: I, II, III, aV_R, aV_L, and aV_F. Imaginary lines drawn from each of the leads intersect at the center of the heart and form a diagram known as the hexaxial reference system. (See *Hexaxial reference system.*)

An axis that falls between 0 and 90 degrees is considered normal. An axis between 90 and 180 degrees indicates right axis deviation, and one between 0 and –90 degrees indicates left axis deviation. An axis between –180 and –90 degrees indicates extreme axis deviation and is called an indeterminate axis.

ELECTRICAL AXIS DETERMINATION

To determine your patient's electrical axis, use the quadrant method or the degree method.

Quadrant method

The quadrant method, a fast, easy way to plot the heart's axis, involves observing the main deflection of the QRS complex in leads I and aV_F. (See *Quadrant method.*) Lead I indicates whether impulses are moving to the right or left, and lead aV_F indicates whether they're moving up or down.

If the QRS-complex deflection is positive or upright in both leads, the electrical axis is normal. If lead I is upright and lead aV_F points down, left axis deviation exists.

When lead I points down and lead aV_F is upright, right axis deviation exists. Both waves pointing down signal extreme axis deviation.

Degree method

A more precise axis calculation, the degree method provides an exact measurement of the electrical axis. (See *Degree method,* page 190.) It also allows you to determine the axis even if the QRS complex isn't clearly positive or negative in leads I and aV_F. To use this method, follow these steps.

1. Review all six leads, and identify the one that contains either the smallest QRS complex or the complex with

Quadrant method

This chart will help you quickly determine the direction of a patient's electrical axis. Observe the deflections of the QRS complexes in leads I and aV$_F$. Then check the chart to determine whether the patient's axis is normal or has a left, right, or extreme axis deviation.

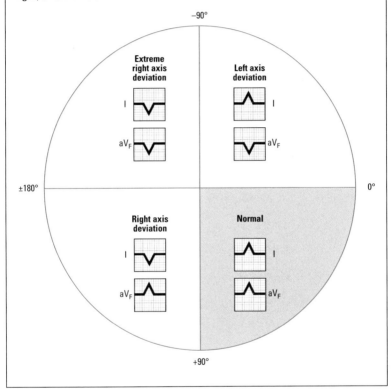

an equal deflection above and below the baseline.

2. Use the hexaxial diagram to identify the lead perpendicular to this lead. For example, if lead I has the smallest QRS complex, then the lead perpendicular to the line representing lead I would be lead aV$_F$.

3. After you've identified the perpendicular lead, examine its QRS complex. If the electrical activity is moving toward the positive pole of a lead, the QRS complex deflects upward. If it's moving away from the positive pole of a lead, the QRS complex deflects downward.

4. Plot this information on the hexaxial diagram to determine the direction of the electrical axis.

Degree method

The degree method of determining axis deviation allows you to identify a patient's electrical axis by degrees on the hexaxial system, not just by quadrant. To use this method, take the following steps.

Step 1
Identify the limb lead with the smallest QRS complex or the equiphasic QRS complex. In this example, it's lead III.

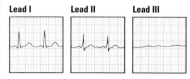

Lead I Lead II Lead III Lead aV$_R$ Lead aV$_L$ Lead aV$_F$

Step 2
Locate the axis for lead III on the hexaxial diagram. Then find the axis perpendicular to it, which is the axis for lead aV$_R$.

Step 3
Now, examine the QRS complex in lead aV$_R$, noting whether the deflection is positive or negative. As you can see, the QRS complex for this lead is negative, indicating that the current is moving toward the negative pole of aV$_R$, which is in the right lower quadrant at +30 degrees on the hexaxial diagram. So the electrical axis here is normal at +30 degrees.

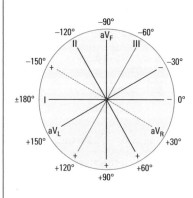

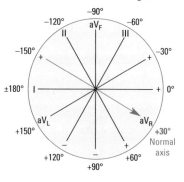

AXIS DEVIATION
Finding a patient's electrical axis can help confirm a diagnosis or narrow the range of possible diagnoses. Factors that influence the location of the axis include the heart's position in the chest, the heart's size, the patient's body size or type, the conduction pathways, and the force of the electrical impulses being generated. Causes of left axis deviation include:

■ normal variation

- inferior wall MI
- left anterior hemiblock
- Wolff-Parkinson-White (WPW) syndrome
- mechanical shifts (ascites, pregnancy, tumors)
- left bundle-branch block (LBBB)
- left ventricular hypertrophy (LVH)
- aging.

Causes of right axis deviation include:

- normal variation
- lateral wall MI
- left posterior hemiblock
- right bundle-branch block (RBBB)
- emphysema
- right ventricular hypertrophy (RVH).

Remember that electrical activity in the heart swings away from areas of damage or necrosis, so the damaged part of the heart will be the last area depolarized. For example, in RBBB, the impulse travels quickly down the normal left side and then moves slowly down the right side. This shifts the electrical forces to the right, causing right axis deviation.

Axis deviation isn't always clinically significant, and it isn't always cardiac in origin. For example, infants and children normally have right axis deviation. Pregnant women normally have left axis deviation.

Disorders affecting 12-lead ECGs

A 12-lead ECG is used to assist in the diagnosis of certain conditions such as angina, Prinzmetal's variant angina, MI, bundle-branch block, pericarditis,

and LVH. By reviewing sample ECGs, you'll know the classic signs to look for. This section examines ECG characteristics of each of these cardiac conditions.

Angina

During an episode of angina, the myocardium demands more oxygen than the coronary arteries can deliver. The arteries can't provide sufficient blood flow, most often as a result of a narrowing of the arteries from coronary artery disease (CAD), a condition that may be complicated by platelet clumping, thrombus formation, and vasospasm. An episode of angina usually lasts between 2 and 10 minutes. The closer to 30 minutes the pain lasts, the more likely it's from MI rather than angina.

The term stable angina has been applied to certain conditions and unstable angina applied to others. In stable angina, pain is triggered by exertion or stress and is typically relieved by rest. Each episode follows the same pattern. Unstable angina, on the other hand, is more easily provoked, commonly waking the patient. It's also unpredictable and worsens over time. The patient with unstable angina is treated as a medical emergency because its onset usually portends an MI.

In addition to the ECG changes noted here, the patient with unstable angina will complain of chest pain that may or may not radiate. The pain is generally more intense and lasts longer than the pain of stable angina. The patient's skin may also be pale and clammy and he may feel nauseous and anxious.

ECG changes associated with angina

Illustrated below are some classic ECG changes involving the T wave and ST segment that you may see when monitoring a patient with angina.

Peaked T wave	Flattened T wave	T-wave inversion	ST-segment depression with T-wave inversion	ST-segment depression without T-wave inversion
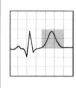	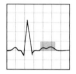	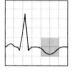	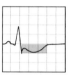	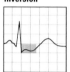

Most patients with either form of angina show ischemic changes on an ECG only during the attack. (See *ECG changes associated with angina*.) Because these changes may be fleeting, always obtain an order for, and perform, a 12-lead ECG as soon as the patient reports chest pain.

The ECG will help you determine which area of the heart and which coronary arteries are involved. By recognizing danger early, you may be able to prevent MI or even death. Drugs are a key component of treating angina and may include nitrates, beta-adrenergic blockers, calcium channel blockers, and aspirin or glycoprotein IIb/IIIa inhibitors to reduce platelet aggregation.

Prinzmetal's variant angina

Prinzmetal's variant angina is a relatively uncommon form of unstable angina. Ischemic pain usually occurs at rest or awakens the patient from sleep.

CAUSES

Prinzmetal's variant angina is caused by a focal episodic spasm of a coronary artery, with or without the presence of an obstructing coronary artery lesion. Cocaine use has also been implicated.

CLINICAL SIGNIFICANCE

Complications include episodes of disabling pain, serious ventricular arrhythmias, atrioventricular (AV) block, MI and, rarely, sudden death.

ECG CHARACTERISTICS

Rhythm: Atrial and ventricular rhythms are normal.
Rate: Atrial and ventricular rates are within normal limits.
P wave: Normal size and configuration.
PR interval: Normal.
QRS complex: Normal.
ST segment: Marked elevation in leads monitoring the heart area where the coronary spasm occurs. This elevation occurs during chest pain and resolves when pain subsides. (See *ECG changes associated with Prinzmetal's angina*.)
T wave: Usually of normal size and configuration.

ECG changes associated with Prinzmetal's angina

This illustration is an example of a 12-lead ECG of a patient with Prinzmetal's angina.

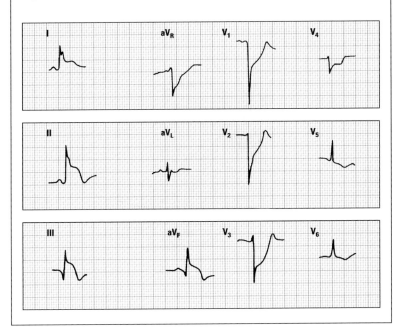

QT interval: Normal.
Other: None.

SIGNS AND SYMPTOMS

A patient with Prinzmetal's angina typically experiences substernal chest pain ranging from a feeling of heaviness to a crushing discomfort, usually while at rest. He may also experience dyspnea, nausea, vomiting, diaphoresis, and arrhythmias.

INTERVENTIONS

Acute management includes the administration of nitroglycerin, which should provide prompt relief from pain by dilating the coronary arteries. For chronic management, long-acting nitrates and calcium channel blockers may be used to help prevent coronary artery spasm. Patients with obstructing coronary artery lesions may benefit from revascularization.

Myocardial infarction

Unlike angina, pain from an MI lasts for at least 20 minutes, may persist for several hours, and is unrelieved by rest.

Reciprocal changes in MI

Ischemia, injury, and infarction—the three I's of myocardial infarction (MI)—produce characteristic ECG changes. The changes shown by leads that reflect electrical activity in damaged areas are shown on the right of the illustration below.

Reciprocal leads, those opposite the damaged area, show opposing ECG changes, as shown to the left of the illustration.

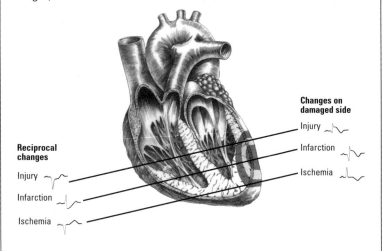

MI usually occurs in the left ventricle, though the location varies depending on the coronary artery affected. For as long as the myocardium is deprived of an oxygen-rich blood supply, an ECG will reflect the three pathologic changes of an MI: ischemia, injury, and infarction. (See *Reciprocal changes in MI*.)

ECG CHARACTERISTICS

The area of myocardial necrosis is called the zone of infarction. Scar tissue eventually replaces the dead tissue, and the damage caused is irreversible. The cardinal ECG change associated with a necrotic area is a pathologic Q wave, which results from lack of depolarization. Such Q waves are permanent. MIs that don't produce Q waves are called non–Q-wave MIs.

The zone of infarction is surrounded by the zone of injury, which shows up on an ECG as an elevated ST segment. ST-segment elevation results from a prolonged lack of blood supply.

The outermost area of the zone of infarction is called the zone of ischemia and results from an interrupted blood supply. This zone is represented on an ECG by T-wave inversion. Changes in the zones of ischemia or injury are reversible.

Generally, as an MI occurs, the patient experiences chest pain, and an ECG will display such changes as ST-segment elevation, which indicates that myocardial injury is occurring. T waves generally flatten and eventually invert.

Rapid treatment can prevent myocardial necrosis. However, if symptoms persist for more than 6 hours, little can be done to prevent necrosis. That's one of the reasons patients are advised to seek medical attention as soon as symptoms begin.

Q waves can appear hours to days after an MI and signify that an entire thickness of the myocardium has become necrotic. Tall R waves in reciprocal leads can also develop. This type of MI is called a transmural, or Q-wave, MI.

Knowing how long such changes last can help you determine how long ago an MI occurred. After the first few days, ST segments return to baseline within 2 weeks. Inverted T waves may persist for several months. Although Q waves don't appear on the ECG of every patient who suffers an MI, when the waves do appear, they remain indefinitely.

INTERVENTIONS

The most important thing you can do for a patient with an MI is to remain vigilant about detecting changes in his condition and ECG. (See *Monitoring MI patients.*)

The primary goal of treatment for an MI is to limit the extent of infarction by decreasing cardiac workload and increasing oxygen supply to the myocardium. Besides rest, pain relief, and supplemental oxygen, such medications as nitroglycerin, morphine sulfate, beta-adrenergic blockers, calcium channel blockers, angiotensin-converting enzyme inhibitors, and antiarrhythmics may be used. Aspirin or glycopro-

---

Monitoring MI patients

Remember that specific leads monitor specific walls of the heart. Here's a quick overview of those leads.
• For an anterior wall myocardial infarction (MI), monitor lead V_1 or MCL_1.
• For a septal wall MI, monitor lead V_1 or MCL_1 to pick up hallmark changes.
• For a lateral wall MI, monitor lead V_6 or MCL_6.
• For an inferior wall MI, monitor lead II.

---

tein IIb/IIIa inhibitors may be used to reduce platelet aggregation. Thrombolytic therapy also may be used to dissolve a thrombus that's occluding a coronary artery.

Other interventions to improve myocardial blood flow include:
- an intra-aortic balloon pump
- percutaneous transluminal angioplasty
- coronary artery atherectomy
- laser treatment
- stent placement
- coronary artery bypass graft.

IDENTIFYING TYPES OF MI

The location of the MI is a critical factor in determining the most appropriate treatment and predicting probable complications. Characteristic ECG changes that occur with each type of MI are localized to the leads overlying the infarction site. (See *Locating myocardial damage,* page 196.) This section takes a look at characteristic ECG changes that occur with different types of MIs.

Locating myocardial damage

After you've noted characteristic lead changes in an acute myocardial infarction, use this chart to identify the areas of damage. Match the lead changes in the second column with the affected wall in the first column and the artery involved in the third column. The fourth column shows reciprocal lead changes.

Wall affected	Leads	Artery involved	Reciprocal changes
Inferior (diaphragmatic)	II, III, aV_F	Right coronary artery	1, aV_L and, possibly, V_4
Lateral	I, aV_L, V_5, V_6	Circumflex artery, branch of left coronary artery	V_1, V_2
Anterior	V_2 to V_4	Left coronary artery, left anterior descending (LAD) artery	II, III, aV_F
Posterior	V_1, V_2	Right coronary artery, circumflex artery	R wave greater than S wave in V_1 and V_2; depressed ST segments; elevated T wave
Anterolateral	I, aV_L, V_4 to V_6	LAD artery, circumflex artery	II, III, aV_F
Anteroseptal	V_1 to V_3	LAD artery	None
Right ventricular	V_4R, V_5R, V_6R	Right coronary artery	None

ANTERIOR WALL MI

The left anterior descending artery supplies blood to the anterior portion of the left ventricle, ventricular septum, and portions of the right and left bundle-branch systems.

When the left anterior descending artery becomes occluded, an anterior wall MI occurs. (See *Recognizing an anterior wall MI.*) Complications include second-degree AV blocks, bundle-branch blocks, ventricular irritability, and left-sided heart failure.

An anterior wall MI causes characteristic ECG changes in leads V_2 to V_4. The precordial leads show poor R-wave progression because the left ventricle can't depolarize normally. ST-segment elevation and T-wave inversion are also present.

The reciprocal leads for the anterior wall are the inferior leads II, III, and aV_F. They show tall R waves and depressed ST segments.

Recognizing an anterior wall MI

This 12-lead ECG shows typical characteristics of an anterior wall myocardial infarction (MI). Note that the R waves don't progress through the precordial leads. Also note the ST-segment elevation in leads V_2 and V_3. As expected, the reciprocal leads II, III, and aV_F show slight ST-segment depression. Axis deviation is normal at + 60 degrees.

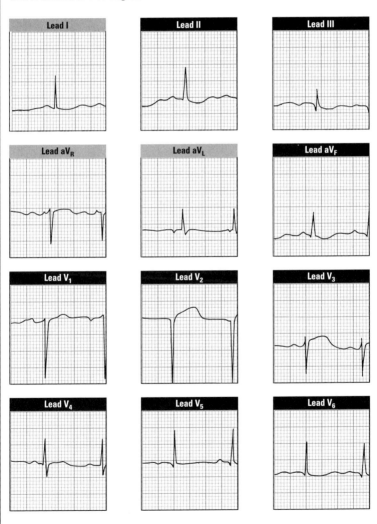

Recognizing an inferior wall MI

This 12-lead ECG shows the characteristic changes of an inferior wall myocardial infarction (MI). In leads II, III, and aV$_F$, note the T-wave inversion, ST-segment elevation, and pathologic Q waves. In leads I and aV$_L$, note the slight ST-segment depression—a reciprocal change. This ECG shows left axis deviation at –60 degrees.

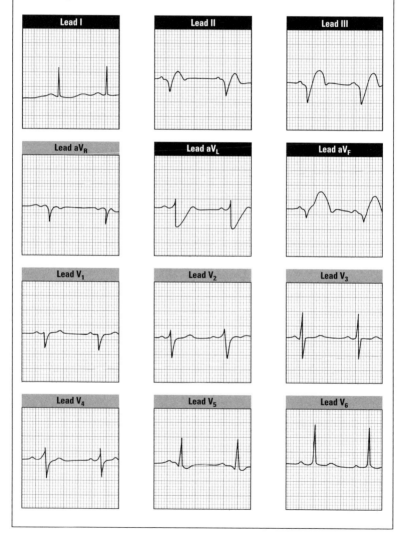

SEPTAL WALL MI

The patient with a septal wall MI is at increased risk for developing a ventricular septal defect. ECG changes are present in leads V_1 and V_2. In those leads, the R wave disappears, the ST segment rises, and the T wave inverts. Because the left anterior descending artery also supplies blood to the ventricular septum, a septal wall MI typically accompanies an anterior wall MI.

LATERAL WALL MI

A lateral wall MI is usually caused by a blockage in the left circumflex artery and shows characteristic changes in the left lateral leads I, aV_L, V_5, and V_6. The reciprocal leads for a lateral wall infarction are leads V_1 and V_2.

A lateral wall MI typically causes premature ventricular contractions (PVCs) and varying degrees of heart block. It usually accompanies an anterior or inferior wall MI.

INFERIOR WALL MI

An inferior wall MI is usually caused by occlusion of the right coronary artery and produces characteristic ECG changes in the inferior leads II, III, and aV_F and reciprocal changes in the lateral leads I and aV_L. (See *Recognizing an inferior wall MI.*) It's also called a diaphragmatic MI because the inferior wall of the heart lies over the diaphragm.

Patients with inferior wall MI are at risk for developing sinus bradycardia, sinus arrest, heart block, and PVCs. This type of MI occurs alone or with a lateral wall or right ventricular MI.

RIGHT VENTRICULAR MI

A right ventricular MI usually follows occlusion of the right coronary artery. This type of MI rarely occurs alone. In 40% of patients, a right ventricular MI accompanies an inferior wall MI.

A right ventricular MI can lead to right ventricular failure. The classic changes are ST-segment elevation, pathologic Q waves, and inverted T waves in the right precordial leads V_2R to V_6R.

Identifying a right ventricular MI is difficult without information from the right precordial leads. If these leads aren't available, you can observe leads II, III, and aV_F or watch leads V_1, V_2, and V_3 for ST-segment elevation. If a right ventricular MI has occurred, use lead II to monitor for further damage.

POSTERIOR WALL MI

A posterior wall MI is caused by occlusion of the right coronary artery or the left circumflex arteries. It produces reciprocal changes in leads V_1 and V_2.

Classic ECG changes for a posterior wall MI include tall R waves, ST-segment depression, and upright T waves. Posterior infarctions usually accompany inferior infarctions. Information about the posterior wall and pathologic Q waves that might occur can be obtained from leads V_7 to V_9, using a posterior ECG.

Bundle-branch block

One potential complication of an MI is bundle-branch block. In this disorder, either the left or the right bundle branch fails to conduct impulses normally. A bundle-branch block that occurs toward the distal end of the left bundle, in the posterior or anterior fasciculus, is called a hemiblock. Some blocks require treatment with a tempo-

Understanding RBBB

In right bundle-branch block (RBBB), the initial impulse activates the interventricular septum from left to right, just as in normal activation (arrow 1). Next, the left bundle branch activates the left ventricle (arrow 2). The impulse then crosses the interventricular septum to activate the right ventricle (arrow 3).

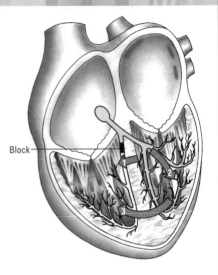

Block

rary pacemaker. Others are monitored only to detect whether they progress to a more complete block.

In a bundle-branch block, the impulse travels down the unaffected bundle branch and then from one myocardial cell to the next to depolarize the ventricle. Because this cell-to-cell conduction progresses much more slowly than along the specialized cells of the conduction system, ventricular depolarization is prolonged.

Prolonged ventricular depolarization means that the QRS complex widens. The normal width is 0.06 to 0.10 second. If it increases to more than 0.12 second, bundle-branch block is present.

After identifying bundle-branch block, examine lead V_1 and lead V_6. You'll use these leads to determine whether the block is in the right or the left bundle branch.

RIGHT BUNDLE-BRANCH BLOCK

RBBB occurs with conditions, such as anterior wall MI, CAD, and pulmonary embolism. It may also occur without cardiac disease. If it develops as heart rate increases, it's called rate-related RBBB. (See *Understanding RBBB.*)

In this disorder, the QRS complex is greater than 0.12 second and has a different configuration, sometimes resembling rabbit ears or the letter "M." (See *Recognizing RBBB.*) Septal depolarization isn't affected in lead V_1, so the initial small R wave remains.

The R wave is followed by an S wave, which represents left ventricular depolarization, and a tall R wave (called R prime, or R′), which represents late right ventricular depolarization. The T wave is negative in this lead; however, the negative deflection

Recognizing RBBB

This 12-lead ECG shows the characteristic changes of right bundle-branch block (RBBB). In lead V_1, note the rsR' pattern and T-wave inversion. In lead V_6, see the widened S wave and the upright T wave. Also note the prolonged QRS complexes.

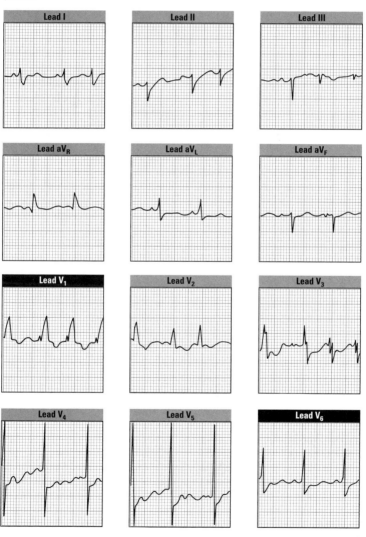

Understanding LBBB

In left bundle-branch block (LBBB), the impulse first travels down the right bundle branch (arrow 1). Then the impulse activates the interventricular septum from right to left (arrow 2), the opposite of normal activation. Finally, the impulse activates the left ventricle (arrow 3).

Block

is called a secondary T-wave change and isn't clinically significant.

The opposite occurs in lead V_6. A small Q wave is followed by depolarization of the left ventricle, which produces a tall R wave. Depolarization of the right ventricle then causes a broad S wave. In lead V_6, the T wave should be positive.

LEFT BUNDLE-BRANCH BLOCK

LBBB never occurs normally. This block is usually caused by hypertensive heart disease, aortic stenosis, degenerative changes of the conduction system, or CAD. (See *Understanding LBBB.*) When it occurs along with an anterior wall MI, it usually signals complete heart block, which requires insertion of a pacemaker.

In LBBB, the QRS complex will be greater than 0.12 second because the

ventricles are activated sequentially, not simultaneously. (See *Recognizing LBBB.*) As the wave of depolarization spreads from the right ventricle to the left, a wide S wave is produced in lead V_1, with a positive T wave. The S wave may be preceded by a Q wave or a small R wave.

In lead V_6, no initial Q wave occurs. A tall, notched R wave, or a slurred one, is produced as the impulse spreads from right to left. This initial positive deflection is a sign of LBBB. The T wave is negative.

It may be difficult to tell the difference between bundle-branch block and WPW syndrome. (See *Distinguishing bundle-branch block from Wolff-Parkinson-White syndrome,* pages 204 and 205.) Whenever you spot bundle-branch block, check for WPW syndrome.

Recognizing LBBB

This 12-lead ECG shows characteristic changes of a left bundle-branch block (LBBB). All leads have prolonged QRS complexes. In lead V_1, note the QS wave pattern. In lead V_6, you'll see the slurred R wave and T-wave inversion. The elevated ST segments and upright T waves in leads V_1 to V_4 are also common in LBBB.

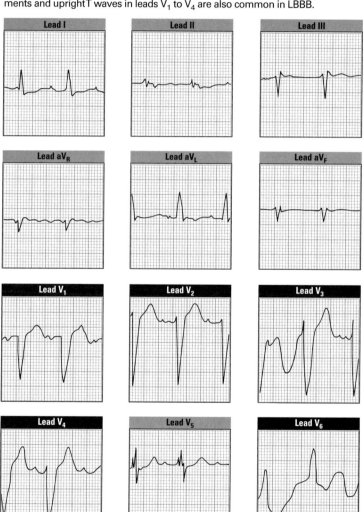

Distinguishing bundle-branch block from Wolff-Parkinson-White syndrome

Wolff-Parkinson-White (WPW) syndrome is a common type of preexcitation syndrome, an abnormal condition in which electrical impulses enter the ventricles from the atria by using an accessory pathway that bypasses the atrioventricular (AV) junction. This results in a short PR interval and a wide QRS complex with an initial slurring of the upward slope of the QRS complex, called a delta wave. Because the delta wave prolongs the QRS complex, its presence may be confused with a bundle-branch block (BBB).

Bundle-branch block

• Carefully examine the QRS complex, noting which part of the complex is widened. A BBB involves a defective conduction of electrical impulses through the right or left bundle branch from the bundle of His to the Purkinje network causing a right or left BBB.

• This conduction disturbance results in an overall increase in QRS duration, or widening of the last part of the QRS complex, while the initial part of the QRS complex commonly appears normal.

• Carefully examine the 12-lead ECG. With BBB, the prolonged duration of the QRS complexes will generally be consistent in all leads.

• Measure the PR interval. BBB has no effect on the PR interval, so the PR intervals are generally normal. Keep in mind, though, that if the patient has a preexisting AV conduction defect, such as first-degree AV block, the PR interval will be prolonged.

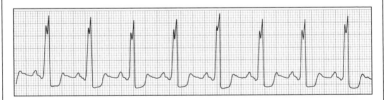

Distinguishing bundle-branch block from Wolff-Parkinson-White syndrome (continued)

Wolff-Parkinson-White syndrome
• A delta wave occurs at the beginning of the QRS complex, usually causing a distinctive slurring or hump in its initial slope. A delta wave isn't present in BBB.

• On the 12-lead ECG, the delta wave will be most pronounced in the leads "looking at" the part of the heart where the accessory pathway is located.
• The delta wave shortens the PR interval in WPW syndrome.

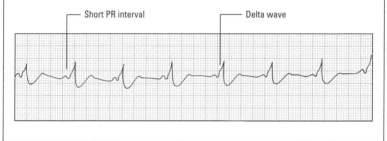

┌─ Short PR interval   ┌─ Delta wave

Pericarditis

Pericarditis is an inflammation of the pericardium, the fibroserous sac that envelops the heart. Pericarditis can be either acute or chronic. The acute form may be fibrinous or effusive, with purulent, serous, or hemorrhagic exudate. Chronic constrictive pericarditis causes dense fibrous thickening of the pericardium.

Possible causes of pericarditis include:
■ viral, bacterial, or fungal disorders
■ rheumatic fever
■ autoimmune disorders
■ complications of cardiac injury.

Regardless of the form, pericarditis can cause cardiac tamponade if fluid accumulates too quickly. It can also cause heart failure if constriction occurs.

ECG CHARACTERISTICS

In pericarditis, ECG changes occur in four stages of disease progression. These changes are secondary to myocardial inflammation and excessive pericardial fluid or a thickened pericardium.

ECG changes evolve through two stages. In the earliest stage, elevation of ST segments accompanies upright T waves. Typically, resolution of the ST-segment elevation marks the beginning of the second stage of acute pericarditis, with widespread T-wave inversion.

The primary ECG abnormality in acute pericarditis is ST-segment elevation. In contrast to the convex ST-segment elevation in acute MI, the ST segments appear somewhat concave in pericarditis. Because pericarditis usually affects the entire myocardial surface, ST segments are usually elevated in

Comparing MI with acute pericarditis

Myocardial infarction (MI) and acute pericarditis cause ST-segment elevation on an ECG. However, the ST segment and T wave (shaded areas) on an MI waveform are quite different from those on the pericarditis waveform.

In addition, because pericarditis involves the surrounding pericardium, several leads will show ST-segment and T-wave changes (typically leads I, II, aV$_F$, and V$_4$ through V$_6$). In MI, however, only those leads reflecting the area of infarction will show the characteristic changes.

These rhythm strips demonstrate the ECG variations between MI and acute pericarditis.

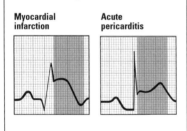

Myocardial infarction   **Acute pericarditis**

most — if not all — leads, except lead aV$_R$. (See *Comparing MI with acute pericarditis.*)
Rhythm: Atrial and ventricular rhythms are usually regular.
Rate: Atrial and ventricular rates usually remain within normal limits.
P wave: Normal size and configuration.
PR interval: Usually normal.
QRS complex: Normal, but a possible decrease in amplitude may occur.
ST segment: In stage 1, the ST segment is elevated 1 to 2 mm in leads II, III,

and aV$_F$ as well as in the precordial leads.
T wave: Remains elevated during the acute phase of pericarditis. As the pericarditis resolves, the T waves become inverted in the leads that had the ST-segment elevation.
QT interval: Normal.
Other: Atrial fibrillation, atrial flutter, or tachycardia may occur as a result of sinoatrial node irritation.

SIGNS AND SYMPTOMS

A patient with acute pericarditis may complain of chest pain, dyspnea, and chills. He may experience fever, diaphoresis, and arrhythmias. A pericardial friction rub is frequently heard. The chest pain typically worsens with deep inspiration and improves when the patient sits up and leans forward.

A patient with chronic pericarditis usually experiences symptoms similar to chronic right-sided heart failure, including edema, ascites, and hepatomegaly.

The most distinctive clinical feature is a palpable, and sometimes audible, sharp knock or rub in early diastole, when the rapidly filling ventricle touches the unexpansive pericardium.

INTERVENTIONS

Acute pericarditis is treated with bed rest and corticosteroids or nonsteroidal anti-inflammatory drugs to relieve pain and inflammation. Infectious pericarditis is treated with antibiotics. Pericardiocentesis is performed for cardiac tamponade, and a complete pericardiectomy may be performed for constrictive pericarditis. Keep in mind that the underlying cause of the pericarditis needs to be identified and treated.

Recognizing left ventricular hypertrophy

Left ventricular hypertrophy (LVH) can lead to heart failure or myocardial infarction. The rhythm strip shown here illustrates key ECG changes of LVH as they occur in selected leads: a large S wave (shaded area below left) in V_1 and a large R wave (shaded area below right) in V_5. If the depth (in mm) of the S wave in V_1 added to the height (in mm) of the R wave in V_5 is greater than 35 mm, then left ventricular hypertrophy is present.

Lead V_1

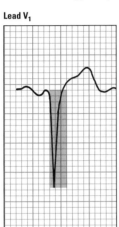

Lead V_5

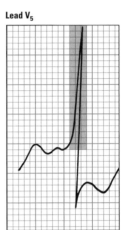

Left ventricular hypertrophy

In LVH, the left ventricular wall thickens. LVH usually results from conditions that cause chronic increases in pressures within the ventricle.

LVH may be caused by mitral insufficiency, cardiomyopathy, aortic stenosis or insufficiency, or systemic hypertension (the most common cause). LVH may lead to left-sided heart failure, which subsequently leads to increased left atrial pressure, pulmonary vascular congestion, and pulmonary arterial hypertension. LVH can decrease coronary artery perfusion, causing MI, or it can alter the papillary muscle, causing mitral insufficiency.

ECG CHARACTERISTICS

Rhythm: Atrial and ventricular rhythms are normal.

Rate: Atrial and ventricular rates are normal.

P wave: May be normal in size and configuration, or may reflect left atrial enlargement.

PR interval: Normal.

QRS complex: May be prolonged or widened with increased amplitude. In lead I, the R wave's amplitude exceeds 1.4 mV. In leads V_1 and V_2, deeper S waves appear. The sum of the S wave

in lead V_1 or V_2 and the R wave in lead V_5 or V_6 exceeds 3.5 mV. The R wave is taller in lead V_6 than in V_5. The R wave's amplitude in lead V_5 or V_6 exceeds 2.6 mV. (See *Recognizing left ventricular hypertrophy,* page 207.)
ST segment: Possibly depressed in the precordial leads when associated with T-wave inversion. This pattern is known as left ventricular hypertrophy with strain.
T wave: May be inverted in leads V_5 and V_6, depending on the degree of hypertrophy.
QT interval: Usually normal.
Other: The axis is usually normal, but left axis deviation may be present.

SIGNS AND SYMPTOMS
Signs and symptoms are related to the underlying disorder.

INTERVENTIONS
Interventions are focused on the management of the underlying disorder such as hypertension.

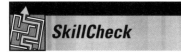
SkillCheck

1. Using the quadrant method of electrical axis determination, a QRS complex with a positive deflection in lead I and a negative deflection in lead aV_F would indicate which of the following axis determinations?
   a. Extreme axis deviation
   b. Left axis deviation
   c. Right axis deviation
   d. Normal axis
Answer: b. Using the quadrant method of electrical axis determination, a QRS complex with a positive deflection in lead I and a negative deflection in lead aV_F indicates left axis deviation.

2. Which of the following conditions is characterized by a prolonged QRS complex, with an rsR′ pattern and T-wave inversion in lead V_1 and a widened S wave and upright T wave in lead V_6?
   a. Right bundle-branch block (RBBB)
   b. Left bundle-branch block
   c. Acute pericarditis
   d. Prinzmetal's angina
Answer: a. RBBB is characterized by a prolonged QRS complex, with an rsR′ pattern and a T-wave inversion in lead V_1 and a widened S wave and upright T wave in lead V_6.

3. The zone of ischemia in the setting of a myocardial infarction (MI) is represented by which of the following changes on an electrocardiogram (ECG)?
   a. Pathologic Q waves
   b. ST-segment elevation
   c. T-wave inversion
   d. Peaked T waves
Answer: c. The zone of ischemia in the setting of a MI is represented by T-wave inversion on the ECG.

4. Which of the following leads reflect the reciprocal leads for the anterior wall?
   a. Leads II, III, and aV_F
   b. Leads I, aV_L, V_5, and V_6
   c. Leads V_2 to V_4
   d. Leads V_1 and V_2
Answer: a. The reciprocal leads for the anterior wall are the inferior leads II, III, and aV_F.

5. Which of the following stages of disease progression in pericarditis coincides with the onset of chest pain and produces ST-segment elevation?

    a. Stage 1
    b. Stage 2
    c. Stage 3
    d. Stage 4

Answer: a. Stage 1 in pericarditis coincides with the onset of chest pain, producing ST-segment elevation.

Appendices, selected references, and index

Appendix A: Quick guide to arrhythmias

Use this chart as a quick reference for identifying characteristics of cardiac arrhythmias. Here are the characteristics of a normal sinus rhythm strip:
- atrial and ventricular rates 60 to 100 beats/minute
- atrial and ventricular rhythms regular
- PR interval of 0.12 to 0.2 second
- QRS duration equal to or less than 0.12 second
- QT interval 0.36 to 0.44 second.

Arrhythmias and features	Causes	Treatment
Sinus arrhythmia • Irregular atrial and ventricular rhythms; corresponds with respiratory cycle • Normal P wave preceding each QRS complex	• A normal variation of sinus rhythm in athletes, children, and older adults • Also seen with digoxin use, morphine use, increased intracranial pressure (ICP), and inferior wall myocardial infarction (MI)	• Typically no treatment is necessary; may correct underlying cause
Sinus tachycardia • Atrial and ventricular rhythms regular • Atrial and ventricular rates are equal; generally 100 to 160 beats/minute • Normal P wave preceding each QRS complex	• Normal physiologic response to fever, exercise, stress, fear, anxiety, pain, dehydration; may also accompany shock, left-sided heart failure, pericarditis, hyperthyroidism, anemia, pulmonary embolism, or sepsis • May also occur with atropine, isoproterenol, aminophylline, dopamine, dobutamine, epinephrine, quinidine, caffeine, alcohol, amphetamine, or nicotine use	• No treatment is necessary if patient is asymptomatic • Correction of underlying cause
Sinus bradycardia • Regular atrial and ventricular rhythms	• Normal during sleep and in a well-conditioned heart such as in an athlete	• No treatment necessary if patient is asymptomatic; if drugs are the cause, may need to discontinue use

Arrhythmias and features	Causes	Treatment
Sinus bradycardia *(continued)* • Rate less than 60 beats/minute • Normal P wave preceding each QRS complex	• Increased ICP; Valsalva's maneuver, carotid sinus massage, vomiting, hypothyroidism; hyperkalemia, hypothermia, cardiomyopathy, or inferior wall MI • May also occur with beta-adrenergic blockers, calcium channel blockers, lithium, sotalol, amiodarone, digoxin, or quinidine use	• For low cardiac output, dizziness, weakness, altered level of consciousness, or low blood pressure: atropine • Temporary pacemaker or permanent pacemaker if condition becomes chronic
Sinus arrest • Atrial and ventricular rhythms normal except for missing complex • Normal P wave preceding each QRS complex	• Coronary artery disease (CAD), acute myocarditis, or acute inferior wall MI • Increased vagal tone as occurs with Valsalva's maneuver, carotid sinus massage, or vomiting • Digoxin, quinidine, procainamide and salicylates, especially if given at toxic levels • Excessive doses of beta-adrenergic blockers, such as metoprolol and propranolol • Sinus node disease	• No treatment necessary if patient is asymptomatic • For mild symptoms, may stop medications that contribute to arrhythmia • If symptomatic, administer atropine • Temporary or permanent pacemaker for repeated episodes
Premature atrial contraction (PAC) • Premature, abnormal-looking P waves, differing in configuration from normal P waves • QRS complexes after P waves, except in blocked PACs • P wave commonly buried in the preceding T wave or identified in the preceding T wave	• In normal heart triggered by alcohol, cigarettes, anxiety, fever, and infectious disease • Heart failure, coronary or valvular heart disease, acute respiratory failure, chronic obstructive pulmonary disease (COPD), electrolyte imbalance, or hypoxia • Digoxin toxicity	• No treatment necessary if patient is asymptomatic • If frequent, may treat with digoxin, procainamide or verapamil • Treatment of underlying cause; patient may need to avoid caffeine or smoking and learn stress reduction measures

(continued)

Arrhythmias and features	Causes	Treatment
Atrial tachycardia • Atrial and ventricular rhythms regular when block is constant; irregular when it isn't • Heart rate 150 to 250 beats/minute • P waves regular but hidden in preceding T wave; precede QRS complexes • Sudden onset and termination of arrhythmia	• Physical or psychological stress, hypoxia, electrolyte imbalances, cardiomyopathy, congenital anomalies, MI, valvular disease, Wolff-Parkinson-White syndrome, cor pulmonale, hyperthyroidism, or systemic hypertension • Digoxin toxicity; caffeine, marijuana, or stimulant use	• Vagal stimulation, Valsalva's maneuver, and carotid sinus massage • Treatment priority is decreasing the ventricular response by using a calcium channel blocker, beta-adrenergic blocker, digoxin, and cardioversion; then consider procainamide or amiodarone if each preceding treatment is ineffective in rhythm conversion • If the ejection fraction is less than 40% or the patient is in heart failure, treat with cardioversion or amiodarone
Atrial flutter • Atrial rhythm regular; rate is 250 to 400 beats/minute • Ventricular rhythm variable, depending on degree of atrioventricular (AV) block, rate is usually 60 to 100 beats/minute • Sawtooth P-wave configuration possible (F waves) • QRS complexes uniform in shape but commonly irregular in rate	• Heart failure, severe mitral valve disease, hyperthyroidism, pericardial disease, COPD, systemic arterial hypoxia, and acute MI	• Treatment of underlying cause • Synchronized cardioversion is the treatment of choice • Drug therapy includes digoxin and calcium channel blockers • Ibutilide fumarate may be used to convert recent-onset atrial flutter to sinus rhythm
Atrial fibrillation • Atrial rhythm grossly irregular; atrial rate greater than 400 beats/minute • Ventricular rhythm grossly irregular • QRS complexes of uniform configuration and duration • PR interval indiscernible	• Ischemic heart disease • Hypertension • Heart failure • Valvular heart disease • Diabetes • Alcohol abuse • Thyroid disorders • Rheumatic heart disease • Lung and pleural disorders	• Control ventricular response with such drugs as diltiazem, verapamil, digoxin, and beta-adrenergic blockers • Ibutilide fumarate may be used to convert new-onset atrial fibrillation to sinus rhythm • Quinidine and procainamide can also convert

Arrhythmias and features	Causes	Treatment
Atrial fibrillation *(continued)* • No P waves; replaced by fine fibrillatory waves		atrial fibrillation to normal sinus rhythm, usually after anticoagulation • Synchronized cardioversion is most successful if used within the first 3 days of treatment
Junctional escape rhythm • Atrial and ventricular rhythms regular • Atrial rate 40 to 60 beats/minute • Ventricular rate 40 to 60 beats/minute (60 to 100 beats/minute is accelerated junctional rhythm) • P waves before, hidden in, or after QRS complex; inverted, if visible • PR interval is less than 0.12 second and is measurable only if the P wave comes before the QRS complex • QRS complex configuration and duration normal	• Inferior wall MI, rheumatic heart disease • Digoxin toxicity, sick sinus syndrome, vagal stimulation	• Atropine for symptomatic slow rate • Pacemaker insertion, if refractory to drugs • Discontinuation of digoxin, if appropriate
Premature junctional contractions • Atrial and ventricular rhythms irregular • P waves inverted; may precede, be hidden within, or follow QRS complex • PR interval less than 0.12 second, if P wave precedes QRS complex • QRS complex configuration and duration normal	• Inferior wall MI or ischemia, swelling of the AV junction after surgery, rheumatic heart disease, valvular heart disease, excessive caffeine intake • Digoxin toxicity (most common)	• Correction of underlying cause • Discontinuation of digoxin, if appropriate • May require elimination of caffeine intake
Junctional tachycardia • Atrial rate is 100 to 200 beats/minute;	• Congenital heart disease in children	• Correction of underlying cause

(continued)

Arrhythmias and features	Causes	Treatment
Junctional tachycardia *(continued)* however, P wave may be absent, be hidden in QRS complex, or precede T wave • Ventricular rate is 100 to 200 beats/minute • P wave inverted • QRS complex configuration and duration normal	• Digoxin toxicity • Swelling of the AV junction after heart surgery • Inferior or posterior wall MI or ischemia	• Discontinuation of digoxin, if appropriate
Wandering pacemaker • Atrial and ventricular rhythms are irregular • PR interval varies • P waves change in configuration indicating that impulses may originate in the sinoatrial node, atria, or AV junction	• May be normal in young patients and is common in athletes who have slow heart rates • Rheumatic carditis, increased vagal tone • Digoxin toxicity	• No treatment if patient is asymptomatic • Treatment of underlying cause if patient is symptomatic
First-degree AV block • Atrial and ventricular rhythms regular • PR interval greater than 0.20 second • P wave preceding each QRS complex; QRS complex normal	• May be seen in a healthy person • Myocardial ischemia or infarction, myocarditis, or degenerative heart changes • Digoxin, calcium channel blocker, and beta-adrenergic blocker use	• Cautious use of digoxin • Correction of underlying cause
Type I second-degree AV block Mobitz I (Wenckebach) • Atrial rhythm regular • Ventricular rhythm irregular • Atrial rate exceeds ventricular rate • PR interval progressively, but only slightly, longer with each cycle until QRS complex disappears (dropped beat)	• Inferior wall MI, CAD, rheumatic fever, or vagal stimulation • Digoxin toxicity, beta-adrenergic blockers, calcium channel blockers	• Treatment of underlying cause • Atropine or temporary pacemaker for symptomatic bradycardia • Discontinuation of digoxin, if appropriate

Arrhythmias and features	Causes	Treatment
Type II second-degree AV block Mobitz II • Atrial rhythm regular • Ventricular rhythm regular or irregular, with varying degree of block • QRS complexes periodically absent	• Severe CAD, anterior MI, or degenerative changes in the conduction system • Digoxin toxicity	• Atropine for symptomatic bradycardia • Temporary pacemaker • Discontinuation of digoxin, if appropriate
Third-degree AV block (Complete heart block) • Atrial rhythm regular • Ventricular rhythm slow and regular; if escape rhythm originates in the AV node the rate is 40 to 60 beats/minute, if escape rhythm originates in the Purkinje system the rate is less than 40 beats/minute • No relation between P waves and QRS complexes • PR interval can't be measured • QRS interval normal (originates in the AV node) or wide and bizarre (originates in the Purkinje system)	• Inferior or anterior wall MI, CAD, degenerative changes in the heart, congenital abnormality, hypoxia, surgical injury • Digoxin toxicity, calcium channel blockers, beta-adrenergic blockers	• Atropine for symptomatic bradycardia • Temporary or permanent pacemaker
Premature ventricular contraction (PVC) • Atrial rate regular in the underlying rhythm; P wave is absent with the premature beat • Ventricular rate irregular during PVC; underlying rhythm may be regular • QRS complex premature, usually followed by a complete compensatory pause • QRS complex wide and bizarre, usually	• Heart failure; myocardial ischemia, infarction, or contusion; myocarditis, myocardial irritation by ventricular catheter such as a pacemaker; hypokalemia metabolic acidosis; or hypocalcemia • Drug intoxication, particularly with cocaine, tricyclic antidepressants, and amphetamines • Caffeine, tobacco, or alcohol use	• If symptomatic, administer procainamide • Treatment of underlying cause • Discontinuation of drug causing toxicity • Potassium chloride I.V. if induced by hypokalemia

(continued)

Arrhythmias and features	Causes	Treatment
Premature ventricular contraction (PVC) *(continued)* greater than 0.12 second in the premature beat • Premature QRS complexes occurring singly, in pairs, or in threes; alternating with normal beats; focus from one or more sites • Most ominous when clustered, multifocal, with R wave on T pattern	• Psychological stress, anxiety, pain, or exercise	
Ventricular tachycardia • Ventricular rate 100 to 200 beats/minute, rhythm is regular or irregular • QRS complexes wide, bizarre, and independent of P waves; duration is greater than 0.12 second • P waves not discernible • May start and stop suddenly	• Myocardial ischemia or infarction, CAD, valvular heart disease, heart failure, cardiomyopathy, ventricular catheters, hypokalemia, hypercalcemia, or pulmonary embolism • Digoxin, procainamide, quinidine, or cocaine toxicity • Anxiety	• If patient is pulseless, immediate cardioversion and resuscitation • If monomorphic ventricular tachycardia, procainamide is given to try to correct the rhythm disturbance; then other drugs, such as amiodarone, are used • If polymorphic ventricular tachycardia, a beta-adrenergic blocker, amiodarone, or procainamide may be given • If patient develops recurrent episodes of ventricular tachycardia unresponsive to drug therapy, may have a cardioverter-defibrillator implanted
Ventricular fibrillation • Ventricular rhythm rapid and chaotic • QRS complexes wide and irregular; no visible P waves	• Myocardial ischemia or infarction, untreated ventricular tachycardia, hypokalemia, acid-base imbalances, hyperkalemia, hypercalcemia, electric shock, or severe hypothermia • Digoxin, epinephrine, or quinidine toxicity	• Rapid defibrillation • Epinephrine or vasopressin followed by defibrillation • Consider antiarrhythmics, such as amiodarone or magnesium • Cardiopulmonary resuscitation (CPR) • Treatment of underlying cause

Arrhythmias and features	Causes	Treatment
Asystole • No atrial or ventricular rate or rhythm • No discernible P waves, QRS complexes, or T waves	• Myocardial ischemia or infarction, heart failure, prolonged hypoxemia, severe electrolyte disturbances such as hyperkalemia, severe acid-base disturbances, electric shock, ventricular arrhythmias, AV block, pulmonary embolism, or cardiac tamponade • Cocaine overdose	• CPR, following advanced cardiac life support protocol • Endotracheal intubation • Transcutaneous pacemaker • Treatment of underlying cause • Repeated doses of epinephrine, as ordered

Appendix B: Cardiac drug overview

Drug	Action	Indications	Adverse affects	Special considerations
Adenosine (Adenocard)	• Slows conduction through the atrioventricular (AV) node	• Paroxysmal supraventricular tachycardia (PSVT), including Wolff-Parkinson-White syndrome	• Chest pain • Dyspnea • Flushing • Transient sinus bradycardia and ventricular ectopy	• Use cautiously in patients with denervated transplanted hearts. • A brief period of asystole (up to 15 seconds) may occur after rapid administration. • Rapidly follow each dose with a 20-ml saline flush.
Amiodarone hydrochloride (Cordarone)	• Exact mechanism not conclusively determined; principal effect on cardiac tissue is to delay repolarization by prolonging the action potential duration and effective refractory period	• Life-threatening ventricular arrhythmias, such as recurrent ventricular fibrillation and recurrent, hemodynamically unstable ventricular tachycardia	• Adult respiratory distress syndrome • Bradycardia • Exacerbation of arrhythmia • Fever • Heart failure • Hepatotoxicity • Hypotension • Nausea and vomiting • Ophthalmic abnormalities may progress to permanent blindness	• Closely monitor patient during loading phase. • Administer doses with meals. • If the patient needs a dosage adjustment, monitor for an extended time because of the long and variable half-life of the drug and the difficulty in predicting the time needed to achieve new steady-state plasma-drug level.
Calcium channel blockers (amlodipine, bepridil hydrochloride, diltiazem hydrochloride, felodipine, isradipine, nicardipine hydrochloride,	• Inhibit influx of calcium through the cell membrane, resulting in a depression of automaticity and conduction velocity in smooth and cardiac muscles • Have different	• Vary for each drug	• Vary among calcium channel blockers; refer to individual drug	• Hypertensive patients treated with calcium channel blockers have a higher risk of myocardial infarction (MI) than patients treated with diuretics or beta-adrenergic blockers. • Abrupt withdrawal may result in increased frequency

220

Drug	Action	Indications	Adverse affects	Special considerations
Calcium channel blockers *(continued)* **nifedipine, nimodipine, nisoldipine, verapamil)**	degrees of selectivity on vascular smooth muscle, myocardium, and conduction and pacemaker tissues			and duration of chest pain. • Monitor cardiac and respiratory function.
Cardiac glycoside (digoxin)	• Increases the force and velocity of myocardial contraction by increasing the refractory period of the AV node	• Slow heart rate in sinus tachycardia from heart failure and control of rapid ventricular contraction rate in patients with atrial fibrillation or flutter	• AV block • Bradycardia • Headaches • Hypokalemia • Nausea and vomiting • Vision disturbances	• Cardiac glycosides are extremely toxic, with a narrow margin of safety between therapeutic range and toxicity. • Vomiting is usually an early sign of drug toxicity. • Discontinue as ordered if patient's pulse rate falls below 60 beats/minute.
Disopyramide phosphate (Norpace)	• Decreases myocardial excitability and conduction velocity; may depress myocardial contractility	• Life-threatening ventricular arrhythmias such as sustained ventricular tachycardia	• Chest pain • First-degree AV block • Hypotension • Nausea • Long QT interval • Shortness of breath • Syncope	• Increases risk of death in patients with non–life-threatening ventricular arrhythmias. • Use with caution in patients with Wolff-Parkinson-White syndrome or bundle branch block.
Flecainide acetate (Tambocor)	• Decreases single and multiple premature ventricular contractions (PVCs) and reduces incidence of ventricular tachycardia • Effect results from a local anesthetic action, especially on the His–Purkinje system in the ventricle	• Sustained ventricular tachycardia • PSVT and atrial fibrillation or flutter	• Dizziness • Dyspnea • Headache • Nausea • Ventricular arrhythmias (new or worsened) • Vision disturbances	• Use cautiously in patients with history of heart failure, MI, or sick sinus syndrome. • Periodically monitor trough plasma levels because 40% is bound to plasma protein. • Increase dosage as ordered at intervals of more than 4 days in patients with renal dysfunction.

(continued)

Drug	Action	Indications	Adverse affects	Special considerations
Ibutilide fumarate (Corvert)	• Delays repolarization by activating a slow, inward current (mostly sodium), which results in prolonged duration of atrial and ventricular action potential and refractoriness	• Rapid conversion of recent-onset atrial fibrillation or atrial flutter	• Nausea • Headache • Torsades de pointes • Worsening ventricular tachycardia	• Stop drug infusion as ordered when arrhythmia stops, if ventricular tachycardia occurs, or if QT interval becomes markedly prolonged.
Lidocaine hydrochloride (Xylocaine)	• Shortens the refractory period and suppresses the automaticity of ectopic foci without affecting conduction of impulses through cardiac tissue	• Acute ventricular arrhythmias	• Dizziness • Hallucinations • Nervousness • Tachycardia • Tachypnea	• Lidocaine doesn't affect blood pressure, cardiac output, or myocardial contractility. • Lidocaine in ineffective against atrial arrhythmias. • Reduce drug dosage as ordered in patients with heart failure or liver disease.
Moricizine hydrochloride (Ethmozine)	• Shortens phase II and III repolarization, leading to decreased duration of the action potential and an effective refractory period	• Life-threatening ventricular arrhythmias such as sustained ventricular tachycardia	• Bradycardia • Dizziness • Headache • Nausea • Sustained ventricular tachycardia	• Use cautiously in patients with sick sinus syndrome because of the possibility of sinus bradycardia, sinus pause, or sinus arrest. • Patient should be hospitalized for initial dosing. • Give before meals because food delays rate of absorption.
Phenytoin sodium (Dilantin)	• Increases the electrical stimulation threshold of heart muscle	• PVCs and tachycardia, especially arrhythmias from digoxin overdose	• Ataxia • Drowsiness • Hepatocellular necrosis (fatal) • Hypotension • Nervousness	• Also used for treatment of chronic epilepsy. • Monitor serum levels. • Abrupt withdrawal may cause status epilepticus. • Use with extreme caution in patients with hypotension or severe myocardial insufficiency.

Drug	Action	Indications	Adverse affects	Special considerations
Procainamide hydrochloride (Procanbid, Pronestyl)	• Produces a direct cardiac effect to prolong the refractory period of the atria and (to a lesser extent) the His–Purkinje system and the ventricles	• Potentially life-threatening ventricular arrhythmias when benefits of treatment clearly outweigh risks	• Diarrhea • Dizziness • Liver failure • Lupus-like syndrome • Nausea and vomiting • Partial or complete heart block	• Increases risk of death in patients with non–life-threatening arrhythmias. • Use with caution in patients with liver or kidney dysfunction. • Tell patient to swallow tablet whole.
Propafenone hydrochloride (Rythmol)	• A class IC antiarrhythmic that reduces inward sodium current in Purkinje and myocardial cells • Decreases excitability, conduction velocity, and automaticity in AV nodal, His–Purkinje, and intraventricular tissue and causes slight but significant prolongation of refractory period in AV nodal tissue	• Life-threatening ventricular arrhythmias, such as ventricular tachycardia, when benefits of treatment outweigh risks	• Constipation • Dizziness • AV block • Headache • Nausea and vomiting • Unusual taste • Ventricular tachycardia	• Monitor liver and renal function studies. • Report any significant widening of QRS complex and any evidence of second- or third-degree AV block. • Increase dosage more gradually as ordered in elderly patients and patients with previous myocardial damage.
Propranolol hydrochloride (Inderal)	• Antiarrhythmic action results from beta-adrenergic receptor block and direct membrane stabilizing action on cardiac cells	• Cardiac arrhythmias, such as ventricular tachycardias, supraventricular arrhythmias, and PVCs	• Bradycardia • Heart failure • Hypotension • Light-headedness • Nausea and vomiting	• Also used for treatment of hypertension, angina pectoris, and MI. • Dosages may differ for hypertension, angina, or MI.
Quinidine sulfate (Quinidex)	• Reduces excitability of the heart and depresses conduction velocity and contractility • Prolongs refractory period and increases conduction time	• Atrial flutter or fibrillation, paroxysmal atrial tachycardia, paroxysmal AV junctional rhythm, and paroxysmal ventricular tachycardia	• Angina-like pain • Complete AV block • Diarrhea • Headache • Hypotension • Light-headedness • Torsades de pointes	• Notify physician immediately if widening QRS complex or increased AV block becomes apparent. • Use with caution in patients who develop a sudden change in blood pressure. • Give with food to minimize GI effects.

(continued)

Drug	Action	Indications	Adverse affects	Special considerations
Tocainide hydrochloride (Tonocard)	• Decreases excitability of cells in the myocardium by decreasing sodium and potassium conductance	• Life-threatening ventricular arrhythmias, including ventricular tachycardia	• Bradycardia • Conduction disorders • Dizziness • Hypotension • Increased ventricular arrhythmias • Left-sided heart failure • Nausea • Pulmonary fibrosis • Tremor	• Use with caution in patients with impaired renal or hepatic function. • Immediately report pulmonary symptoms, such as wheezing, coughing, and dyspnea.
Vasopressin (ADH) Pitressin	• Acts at the renal tubular level to increase cyclic adenosine monophosphate, which in turn increases water permeability at the renal tubule and collecting duct; results in increased urine osmolality and decreased urine flow rate • Also directly stimulates vasoconstriction of capillaries and small arterioles	• Alternative to epinephrine in the treatment of adult shock-refractory ventricular fibrillation; may also provide hemodynamic support in vasodilatory shock by maintaining coronary perfusion pressure	• Tremor • Headache • Vertigo • Vasoconstriction • Arrhythmias • Cardiac arrest • Myocardial ischemia and angina • Decreased cardiac output • Abdominal cramps and flatulence • Nausea and vomiting • Cutaneous gangrene • Water intoxication	• Use with caution in patients with history of cardiovascular disease because drug may provoke cardiac ischemia and angina. • Use extreme caution to avoid extravasation with this drug because of the risk of necrosis and gangrene.

Selected references

Cosio, F.G., and Delpon, E. "New Antiarrhythmic Drugs for Atrial Flutter and Atrial Fibrillation: A Conceptual Breakthrough at Last?" *Circulation* 105(3):276-78, January 2002.

Dubin, D. *Rapid Interpretation of EKGs*, 6th ed. Tampa, Fla.: Cover Publishing Company, 2000.

ECG Cards, 3rd ed. Springhouse, Pa.: Springhouse Corp., 2000.

ECG Interpretation Made Incredibly Easy, 2nd ed. Springhouse, Pa.: Springhouse Corp., 2002.

Faber, T.S., et al. "Impact of Electrocardiogram Recording Format on QT Interval Measurement and QT Dispersion Assessment," *Pacing and Clinical Electrophysiology* 24(12):1739-747, December 2001.

Huikuri, H.V., et al. "Sudden Death Due to Cardiac Arrhythmias," *New England Journal of Medicine* 345(20):1473-482, November 2001.

Landesberg, G., et al. "Perioperative Myocardial Ischemia and Infarction: Identification by Continuous 12-lead Electrocardiogram with Online ST-Segment Monitoring," *Anesthesiology* 96(2):264-70, February 2002.

Mastering ACLS. Springhouse, Pa.: Springhouse Corp., 2002.

McAlister, F.A. "Atrial fibrillation, Shared Decision Making, and the Prevention of Stroke," *Stroke* 33(1):243-44, January 2002.

Wagner, G.S. *Marriott's Practical Electrocardiography*, 10th ed. Philadelphia: Lippincott Williams & Wilkins, 2001.

Index

i refers to an illustration; t refers to a table.

i refers to an illustration; t refers to a table.